Praise for *Fierce Medicine*

"*Fierce Medicine* is classic Ana Forrest: straight ahead life tales from one of the meteors of the modern yoga movement . . . laced with the intense focus of a Tiger seeking the freedom of the heart."
—John Friend, founder of Anusara yoga

"Ana Forrest has been a pioneer spirit in excavating the truths of our embodied experience. Like never before, she has courageously opened her life to share her own powerful healing experience through yoga as a way of liberating all beings to follow their own authentic journey of mending the sacred wheel of their life through breath, body, and spirit."
—Shiva Rea, yogini

"Ana Forrest is a phenomenon: Her breathtaking yogic abilities and extraordinary, passionate teaching inspire and challenge people to go continually deeper. Ana's unique journey of triumph over adversities leads people to find strength from within."
—Joel Kramer and Diana Alstad, coauthors of
The Passionate Mind Revisited and *The Guru Papers*

"I was lucky to have had Ana Forrest introduce me to the yoga experience many years ago. It transformed my life in such a positive way that I can suggest here that should the reader not be able to attend a 'live' session with Ana, getting into *Fierce Medicine* would definitely be the next best thing."
—Jerry Moss, cofounder of A&M Records

"This woman saved my life. She saves it every day when I step on the mat for my Forrest Yoga practice and her book is a sacred offering from her fiercely creative heart that challenges us to not only survive the worst, but to find the path to being fully, passionately alive. My path has so far taken me from being a counter-weapons of mass destruction planner for the US Air Force, to life as a USAF spouse, Forrest Yoga teacher, and Forrest Yoga liaison to the military; her words inspire me to revel in my work as a way to honor the voice of my Spirit. That work is now to bring her wisdom to my tribe, my people—our nation's warriors. They need and deserve to walk the healing road that this book offers. Ana's stories of courage, commitment, and resilience resonate with the warrior heart beating its powerful drum inside us all."

—Elizabeth Pope, Forrest yoga teacher

FIERCE MEDICINE

Breakthrough Practices
to Heal the Body
and Ignite the Spirit

ANA T. FORREST

HarperOne
An Imprint of HarperCollins*Publishers*

HarperOne

Please consult with your medical provider before beginning any exercise program.

HarperCollins books may be purchased for educational, business, or sales promotional use. For information please write: Special Markets Department, HarperCollins Publishers, 10 East 53rd Street, New York, NY 10022.

HarperCollins website: http://www.harpercollins.com

HarperCollins®, 📖®, and HarperOne™ are trademarks of HarperCollins Publishers

FIRST EDITION

Photography by Nils Vidstrand

Library Of Congress Cataloging-In-Publication Data

Forrest, Ana T.
 Fierce medicine : breakthrough practices to heal the body and ignite the spirit / by Ana T. Forrest. — 1st ed.
   p. cm.
 ISBN 978–0–06–186424–7
 1. Yoga. I. Title.
 RA781.7.F675 2011
 613.7'046—dc22   2010048615

11 12 13 14 15 RRD(H) 10 9 8 7 6 5 4 3

Dedication

This is dedicated to the people who gave me a compelling reason to live and, most important, who first taught me how to love: my students.

To the people who connected to how precious Forrest Yoga and Mending the Hoop of the People are to me and who now help spread this teaching in the world: my Forrest Yoga teachers.

To the people who have pledged to be the Guardians of the legacy of Forrest Yoga and to continue to educate the Forrest Yoga teachers and students long after I die: Kelley Rush, Colleen Millen, Heidi Sormaz, Ann Hyde, Christine Raffa, Brian Campbell, Sinhee McCabe, Suzi Zobrist, Steve Emmerman, Bridget Foley, Panther Cat (Catherine) Allen, Erica Mather, Cheryl Deer, Talya Ring.

To the people who have helped move me or my book forward in life: Nick Angelakos, Morris Netherton, Heyoka Merrifield, Debbie Finley-Justus, Brooke Medicine-Eagle, Arwin Dreamwalker-Larkin, Tom Yellowtail, Rosalyn Bruyere, Eric Perret, Linda Loewenthal, Cindy DiTiberio and all the people at HarperOne, Betsy (Elizabeth) Rapoport, Lynann Politte, Panther Cat (Catherine) Allen, Maria Pappas, Susan Missner, Rani Kamaruddin, Michael Metzler, Ellen Heed, Bonnie Argo, Dr. LeRoy R. Perry, and Gary Karten.

Ana's Prayer

Sacred Ones, how can we dance with what is immovable in our lives? Help us to weave our life into a masterpiece. Help us to use our healing breath to bring new life to cell tissue so our cells reorganize in a healthy way. I pray we learn how to make the dream of our life come true, knowing that we must be flexible and quick enough on our feet to accommodate how our life changes as the dream comes into being. I will dance with the dreams I have for this book in ways I can't conceive of yet, but I pray that I'll be quick afoot enough to dance in beauty with it. Aho!

CONTENTS

INTRODUCTION

RAGING THUNDER, crackling lightning, and ferocious winds have followed me throughout my life. And I'm not just talking about high-energy weather disturbances, but the abuse that drove me to alcohol by age four, cigarettes by age six, weed and pills a few years later, and the raging storms inside my body: epilepsy, migraines, paralysis, and bulimia. Those storms ravaged me, left marks deep inside me, until I figured out how to use them to scour myself clean and turn their energy toward my own healing. I learned to give voice to the truths of the thunder and lightning within my body and spirit.

Now I understand that some of my gifts are to induce cataclysm and to be a Truth Speaker—someone who is committed to speaking about difficult and hidden things, to revealing the beauty in the world in order to teach and heal. In seeking to heal myself, I had to first learn to surf all that violent, chaotic energy in my own life. I discovered that I was a pathfinder to other people's truths, that I could help them navigate the storms in their lives and seek a way out of pain. My soul's work is to guide other people through dramatic transformations.

My quest for the teachers and the tools that would help me on my path has taken me to the great masters of India, to caves in the Himalayas, and to Native American Medicine circles. To see whether the wild promises held true, I sought out and mastered nearly every advanced, freaky, esoteric practice the ancient sutras and the healing arts had to offer. I have no loyalty to concepts that aren't *true* for me. Although I studied Yoga with B. K. S. Iyengar himself, the most important lesson I learned from him was to disobey the dictator if you don't find a man's character congruent with his teachings. I learned more about true healing and wisdom from a humble woman who ministered to the poor of India and from that country's *sadhus*—wild and saintly women and men—than I did from people with outsized reputations and followings. I spent almost six years on a Native American reservation where I first learned to call the storms my friends. Training as a Pipe Carrier and Medicine Woman, I learned the power of ceremony. I studied energetic healing techniques with internationally acclaimed Medicine Woman and healer Rosalyn Bruyere. I discarded what didn't work from both ancient and modern wisdom traditions and braided in the wisdom from my years as a horse whisperer to create the unique approach I call Forrest Yoga. I have been learning and teaching Yoga for more than thirty-six years. What I present here are tools for life transformation, forged in the cauldron of my own experience and tested on the hundreds of thousands of students I've taught in that time.

This book lays out a system of practices founded in Yoga and Native American Medicine. This system specifically addresses the challenges and stresses—physical, emotional, mental, and spiritual—that *all* people face. The Lakota Medicine Man Black Elk lived through the shattering of the spine of his people. Describing the desperate spiritual bereftness he saw around him, he said, "The Rainbow Hoop of the People has been broken." The Rainbow Hoop refers to people living harmoniously just as the colors of the rainbow lie side by side. The People he speaks of include the other inhabitants of the earth, including the animals. I created Forrest Yoga to do my part in Mending the Hoop of the People. This is my life's calling, my Spirit Pledge.

A lot of people come to Forrest Yoga because they've got a storm brewing inside them. Many are in pain—although sometimes they don't even recognize what kind of pain. They've tried numbing out with food or TV or sex or work or alcohol or drugs, and they want to find a different way. Others come because they don't feel *anything*—boy are we good at numbing ourselves out—and they want to live inside their bodies again. Still others come because they want to connect or reconnect with a deeper part of themselves—a yearning they haven't even learned to name or articulate. (Of course, some come because they want a Christy Turlington Yoga butt, and I help them too.) The first thing I do is help all these people learn to listen to what their bodies are trying to tell them.

This is the work I do: help people recognize those moments when the body speaks from a deeply profound level, then guide them in getting the work done through growing, healing, and evolving. The transformations are often dramatic, and though the details change, I've seen personal revolutions happen.

Growth often starts in quantum leaps, and these are precious, often terrifying moments. When that leap presents itself, can you recognize it? Are you willing to take it? The sweetness of midwifing that kind of transformation is what continues to fuel me. It's why I'm writing this book.

Although our struggles are unique, each of us dances with many of the same monsters: fear, pain, resistance to change, collapse in the face of failure, reluctance to open the heart. I've tangoed more than a few times with each of these soul-twisters—I'm dancing still—so in each chapter I'll share my own story and what I've learned from it, how I've used my lessons to help others through the same difficult places, and how you can apply them right now.

I've built these lessons around what I call a Spiritual Focus and a Physical Focus. These aren't quick-fix platitudes and pretty postures (because, as Sun Bear, one of the elders on the Washington reservation, used to say: "If it don't grow corn, it ain't worth shit"). They are specific spiritual and physical exercises that anyone can engage in, so long as they're willing to put in the work.

I've shared my story with my students, and I share it here in this book because although the details differ, most of us are looking for the same thing: not just healing, but a connection to something greater than ourselves. I call it Spirit. Now that I've tasted the sweetness of my own connection to Spirit, I want to embody it, walk its path, and show you how to do the same. Doing this requires uncovering and feeling through the experiences long buried within our bodies so the traumas can clear, and it involves reexamining the decisions we have made from our fear and trauma. This work can help us digest our experiences and glean wisdom from them. Our bodies tell our stories, and they always tell the truth when we listen. I want to help you hear your body's story and then teach it to speak its truth.

I teach my own unique system of Yoga—but more importantly, I teach how to use the discerning awareness that comes with Yoga in a way that brings healing to the body and the spirit, and ultimately helps people take control and power over their own lives—and then, perhaps most importantly, design the lives they want to live. I hope this book will help you not only heal, but also recognize what fills you up, what nourishes you. I hope it will help you mend your own hoop and learn to give from a place of fullness.

According to Native American tradition, from which I've received so much wisdom and inspiration, *Beauty* with a capital *B* refers to a very specific perception of the world, one informed by elegant balance and harmony. To walk in Beauty is one of the guidelines for living a life correctly. I believe that each of us is responsible for and capable of walking the path that our Spirit dictates. That is walking in Beauty. If you want this in your life, you can learn to listen to your Spirit. And begin your walk.

May we all walk in Beauty,
Ana Tiger Forrest

1

STALKING FEAR:
FROM PREY TO PREDATOR

THEY TELL ME I was born crippled, a funny-looking kid, my feet and the left side of my body all twisted. Family lore is that the doctor had told my mother that they would have to break all the bones in the left side of my body and then put me in a full-body cast. Luckily, we had a relative who was a chiropractor, which back in the fifties, was like having a witch doctor in the family. He told my mother, "Her bones are soft; you can straighten them out."

My earliest memory is of Mother's hands coming through the bars of my crib, and the terror and pain as she twisted my feet and legs this way and that, again and again. Whatever she was doing to me in the crib was probably her attempt to follow my relative's instructions. It must have worked; the next time Mother took me to the pediatrician, there was no more talk of breaking bones and setting body casts. The doctor, without even glancing at any notes or file, just waved her away: "See, I told you she'd be fine."

Fine, perhaps, but certainly not fixed. I crawled as much as possible as a babe, since it was so hard to walk and I looked so weird doing it. When I was five or six, my mother forced me to wear heavy orthopedic shoes fitted with steel braces inside that made walking even more difficult.

Every day I was supposed to shuffle along a chart she laid down on the floor. The chart was dotted with footprints where I was supposed to step—a kind of evil Twister game. The steel braces raised blisters and welts on my feet, and the daily therapy made them bleed. God, I hated those shoes. Once I tried burning them in the fireplace—the damn steel braces wouldn't burn. That earned me a smack from my mother.

Nothing new about that. Our home was a terrifying place where I never felt safe. From the outside, our lives must have looked pretty normal. We lived in a California tract house, fairly new, with four bedrooms and two baths for five people: my mother, my dad, my older brother and sister, and me. Inside, though, things had gone to hell. My father had long since moved into a separate bedroom. The house was always filthy and foul-smelling, with crusted dishes piled up in the sink, ants everywhere, dried cat scat in the corners and under the couches. My morbidly obese brother hoarded food, especially after a padlock appeared on the refrigerator door, so odd smells came from his room too.

My mother, who was also obese, was always hitting me for some reason or another. She could switch in a moment—from a helpless, whining hypochondriac to a violent, out-of-control tyrant. The smallest infraction—or sometimes nothing at all—would start her on a rant, which often escalated into slapping and coming after me. "Demon seed," she'd say, or "bad seed," or "goddamn kid"—she would scream at me.

She'd go off on my brother too—I don't remember if my sister was ever in her sights—but I was her favorite target. I don't know why. Maybe trying to fix my funky feet and legs wore her out and made her sick of me. Maybe she was just exhausted and frustrated trying to be a mother to three young children. Maybe she was just nuts. All I knew was that whenever I was home, I was afraid of her. She was a hammersmith's daughter and had a hell of a swing.

In the beginning, I'd beg her to stop, but after a few years, I stopped protesting, even stopped crying—I refused to give her that much, to show her I was broken. I also discovered a method of protecting myself from her rages. Whenever my mother went on a rampage, I'd run to my bedroom closet, pull myself up onto a high shelf, and tuck myself behind the clothes and boxes, trembling. There in the dark, I'd close my eyes and just . . . disappear. I'd hear her tearing around my room, tossing aside clothes and shoes, looking behind furniture. I was mere feet away, but she'd never find my hiding place. I'd somehow figured out how to extinguish my life force so she couldn't track me. It worked every time.

School was safe enough—inside the classroom. But getting there and back was a nightmare. An undersized, pale, sickly kid with bruised eyes and funny-looking clunky shoes, I had an obvious target on my back. The kids would circle me, calling me strange names, like "Jew bitch with nigger socks." (I had no idea where they got this or what it meant.) The worst bully was my neighbor. It wasn't like I could avoid her; we lived on a dead-end street, and I had to walk by her house to get to school. One day she dragged me into her backyard, picked up a board studded with nails and waved it at my head, laughing as her growling German shepherd menaced me, jaws snapping.

My waking hours were ruled by fear, yet sleep was no relief. That's when the sharks and other shadowy monsters stalked me. People tell me you can't die in your dreams, but I died a thousand deaths—torn limb from limb by sharks and demons, crushed slowly by stones, drowned, sucked into tsunamis. Whenever I finally succumbed to sleep, I lay pinned to my bed, paralyzed by these horrific apparitions. The next morning I'd wake up sore, covered with bruises, sometimes with ripping pain in my intestines and butt. The pain came on with such suddenness, such violence, that I'd gasp. Sometimes I'd force myself to stay awake for days rather than surrender to such dreadful dreams.

But I was a creative kid, and when I was about four, I figured out one way to numb myself to the constant fear: raid the liquor cabinet. I remember walking on my pathetic legs to get there. I snuck out to the kitchen and squatted near the cabinet. I unscrewed the caps and stole sips from the caramel brown bottles full of something that was sickly sweet, the pretty emerald green liquor, the clear bottles with the stuff that burned on the way down, the squarish bottle with the red waxy seal and sweet amber fluid. It wasn't that I liked the taste so much; I liked the strange fiery sensation on my tongue, the feeling of floating away from my body. I liked that it altered my filthy reality very quickly. The fear was still there, but it wasn't as sharp.

Then, about two years later, I finally found a safe haven, an escape hatch away from the horrors of home and the torment of the neighborhood bullies: a horse stable. For as long as I can remember, I've shared a sacred bond with horses. I've been told that someone had taken me to a parade when I was a year old, and there I'd seen my first horse. I'd pointed and said, "I want." I was about six when my mother started taking me to a rent stable a few miles from home. I'm not even sure why she took me; probably just to get me out of her hair.

Pretty soon that broken-down rent stable, Azusa Canyon Stables, became my real home. It wasn't a fancy place, just a bunch of horses for hire, some boarding. The owner, a rasty, amazing Greek Jew named Nick Angelakos, was a real wild man, though. When he was younger, he used to jump his horses through rings of fire at the circus, or over a jalopy with a bunch of smiling passengers. He had framed photos of his circus escapades all over his office, and I couldn't stop staring at them. Nick was pretty fearless, and he didn't condone fear in animals or children. I was at least a foot shorter and five or six years younger than anyone else working there, but he must have seen something in me that I didn't yet see in myself. Pretty soon we had a deal: I'd help out at the stables, and he'd teach me to ride. For the next six years, I did whatever I could to be around those horses: mucking stalls, leading groups of riders, and eventually training horses.

I learned a lot about facing my fears by working with those horses. Far from being gentle souls, horses will bully each other, and they'll bully humans. I was always getting stepped on and pushed over and kicked. Since I was such a runt, I really had to learn how to make those huge animals pay attention, let them know, "I may be short, but you better know I'm here." When they'd rear up or try to kick or bite me, I refused to be spooked. Instead, I faced them down, drawing my tiny body up as tall as I could, keeping my voice low and determined. "Oh, no you don't. You're coming with me right now." I got kicked to pieces a million times, but I stopped being afraid of getting stomped. Size has nothing to do with standing up to someone. I began to grow my power.

I remember the moment I knew for sure that I'd changed my relationship with fear. My mother and I were carrying a heavy piece of wooden furniture down the hallway when I accidentally dropped my end. "Demon seed!" she screamed at me. "Evil!" She brought back her arm to do her usual routine. But by this time I was close to twelve, much stronger from working at the stable. I'd been dealing with fifteen hundred pounds of equine temper often enough that I found myself thinking, *This is just a two-legged one, and a fat one at that.* On that day, I reached out and caught her hammersmith's fist mid-swing. There were no words, just the two of us staring straight into each other's eyes and a realization: this ends it. Fear left me and infected her. I think she was as astonished as I was. She struggled for a moment and then let her arm fall. She pretty much quit going after me after that.

That was a turning point for me. I learned to do a switch—instead of running from the fear, I turned around and went after it, making it my ally. On the playground, I challenged the toughest bully to take her best shot. "Go ahead, hit me!" I kept backing her down, right in front of her posse. I don't know whether she was scared or just confused, but she kept her distance from then on.

I was done living in fear. I took a pledge to stop being prey, to turn around, face my fear, and stalk it. I've lived that way ever since.

FEAR TRAINING

I started deliberately doing things that terrified me; I called it fear training. As a teenager, I was afraid of being out in the desert—it was so dry, so exposed to the elements. So I ran off to Hesperia in the Mojave Desert in Southern California to take my first job training horses on my own. When I first arrived, I felt like I'd been plunked down on the lifeless surface of the moon: blazing heat, no water. Gradually I learned to walk through the heat the way you'd ford a river—loose-limbed, going with the flow. I discovered an incredible amount of beauty and life in the desert; it was just subtler than I was used to. You have to look closer, but then you see hares, mice, rattlesnakes, buzzards, hawks, and all the folks that live in the desert. I began to sense the desert's rhythms, the way the flowers can carpet the land after a cloudburst and then three days later leave just seeds rolling across the dry earth. The very briefness of those flowers' lives added to the poignancy of it. I began to love what I had feared.

A few years later, when I lived up in the Santa Barbara Forest in my early twenties, I decided to stalk my fear of heights. I'd perch on this tiny ledge high above a river filled with rocks. I'd stand there, at least twenty or twenty-five feet above the water, petrified, waiting for the fear to leave. But it never did—so I would jump anyway. I'd keep climbing up that ledge and jumping off five or six times, even though my heart hammered harshly in my chest. I realized the fear wasn't going to go away, but my paralysis within the fear would.

Sometimes I'd hesitate. I had this paradigm in my head: *If I just stand here long enough, the fear will go away and I'll jump and I'll be fearless.* That didn't happen. I discovered instead how not to be stopped by my fear. I tried stilling my fear by sitting down and breathing deeply, but that really wasn't all that helpful. After a while, I'd clamber all the way up and just jump right away so the fear wouldn't have time to build, the paralysis wouldn't deepen, and all the subterranean scary stories in my head couldn't bubble up. I didn't wait to feed the fear. I just took a deep breath, exhaled, and jumped. The fear was there, but it wasn't unmanageable. I'd believed that in order to do what I was afraid of, I had to get rid of the fear first, but that turned out to be only an idea, not the truth. You have to do something two hundred times before the fear will disperse. Are you still afraid of something? Just do it again. Do it again. Do it again.

Maybe I couldn't banish all my fears, but I made the choice to stop allowing them to rule my life.

CHOOSING THE BRAVE-HEARTED PATH

It takes a lot of courage to explore your fear. Courage isn't the numbed-out, flinty, Clint Eastwood–esque stoicism we're accustomed to, but instead it's daring to experience our feelings—even if this requires painful awakening—with discernment and intelligence. Choose the Brave-Hearted Path: have the courage to truly feel what's going on inside you when you're afraid, and respond appropriately. This requires patience.

Walk the Brave-Hearted Path now by deciding you will no longer be afraid of being afraid. Reframe your fear; be willing to get sick and tired of being sick and tired. I also got sick of being everyone's lunch. Now I refuse: You don't get even a snack from me!

So, right now I want to help you make the choice to face your fears by using Forrest Yoga poses to wash fear and its toxic aftereffects out of your body. I want you to be very grounded in proper technique so that Forrest Yoga can work for you.

SPIRITUAL FOCUS:
EXERCISES FOR WALKING THROUGH THE SPOOK ZONE

There's a saying: *When in fear, or in doubt, run in circles, scream, and shout.*

We have a lot of internal responses to fear. We push it away, we deny it, we freeze, flee, or attack (fight-or-flight syndrome). But there are alternative ways of responding to fear. Imagine your fear as a separate energy—a cat backed into a corner having a hissing fit. You could walk over, sit down next to it, and lean your hip up against this fluffed-up, tense cat—immediately your relationship will change. The cat won't change its internal makeup, but it'll change its fear response to whatever it was hissing about. Still, I wouldn't suggest picking it up and snuggling it until it calms down a little. This fear is a part of you that's scared to death. Go down and comfort it—it's a part of you. It's not something to be beaten down by or to wall off. Studying your fear is such a radically weird activity that it begins to change that part of you that's in fear.

Change your response to fear. Stop numbing out. Track it and learn and grow. Here are my five steps for changing your relationship with fear:

1 Identify the fear

2 Turn around, hunt it, stalk it

3 Stop making decisions based on fear

4 Find the healing within the fear

5 Snuggle up to your fear

IDENTIFY THE FEAR

What exactly are you afraid of, and where did that fear come from? Start working that path of discovery. Fear always has an origin. *Always.* People with anxiety attacks might disagree, but it's true; they just don't know what the origin is yet. Once you find the source of your fear, you can begin to address it.

I had a friend who was afraid of binging and losing control. She found herself Googling the calories in a single M&M. "I'm afraid of an M&M," she told me. "I feel so stupid, but I have this fear that I'll lose control if I eat one." "What would happen then?" I asked her. "I'll eat the whole bag," she said. "What would happen then?" "I'd break the promise to myself and my friend; we're dieting together." My friend was ultimately afraid she'd threaten a precious friendship; that's a painful betrayal. Behind these fears, however, were other fears and self-mutilating thoughts: *I'll never lose the weight. I'm a moron who can't get control over one little M&M.* And behind *those* fears, way deep down, was her most primal fear: *If I'm not slim and sexy, I'm not worthwhile. I'm unlovable, useless; I could be thrown away.* Being cut off from the tribe—that's some pretty scary stuff. So what seemed like the fear of binging was in actuality a lot more complex. Once my friend came to that realization, she could begin to deal with her feelings of unworthiness.

Our bodies archive our life experiences and often tell the stories of our deepest fears. When Dr. Timothy McCall came to one of my Yoga classes, I noticed right away that he had this weird twisty back; he was bent over like a perpetual comma. Where did *that* come from? I had him just breathe and stay in a forward bend, and he suddenly remembered climbing a tree as a young boy when he'd fallen and landed on his head, neck, and upper back. He'd really injured himself. His family freaked out—*Oh my god, he could have broken his neck, been paralyzed for life!* So here was this little boy: hurt, in shock, defenseless, and his parents were pouring out their terror into him. All that loving concern laced with terror made his body kink over and hold this physiological imprint. He'd made it worse by a lifetime of sitting in front of his computer, hunching, writing too many books. His body curled around the experience and never let go until my class, where I started to help him unwind it. It freed his upper back, and his body has been changing radically ever since.

Even though I spent so much time working on my fears as a teenager and a young adult, and even though I could point to my fearful upbringing as a cause, I spent many years feeling fearful, wild, crazy, out of control—and I didn't really understand why. I just had this sense that I hadn't reached the black heart of things. Then one day I was in Dolphin pose, butt up in the air, when I was jolted not just by a memory of hands grabbing my hip and thigh and being brutally raped, but the actual painful feelings. Suddenly all these horrific memory fragments rushed to the surface—all those times I'd woken with intense pain and bruising around my genitals and butt, feeling drugged out and woozy. This wasn't the first time I suspected that I had been sexually abused as a little girl, but it was the moment that I made the decision to turn from prey to predator.

I started gasping for air, shaking uncontrollably, and going numb, but I thought, *Hell no! I'm gonna chase this abuser out of my body!* I went rampaging through my pelvis and colon, looking for every little vestige of fear—hip joints, blood vessels. I could smell the fear, taste it, feel the acidic burn of it. When I came to each painful spot inside my body, I would breathe and fill it with my essence, *will* it back to life. As I'll discuss in a later chapter, it took me years and years of therapy to come to terms with the physical and sexual abuse to which I'd been subjected, and I won't minimize the hard emotional, physical, psychological, and spiritual work involved, but it was the decision that day on the mat to transform from prey to predator that gave me the courage to take that journey.

When I finally stalked the origins of my abuse, I understood why I'd always felt so wild and crazy. Once you stalk the fear back to its source, you can begin to reconcile it. You'll inevitably find your fear ramping up as you hunt—keep going; you're on the right track! If you've suffered any kind of abuse or other trauma, please work with a therapist or other trusted professional as you take this journey.

TURN AROUND, HUNT IT, STALK IT

If you're still not sure what's causing your fear, it's time to go hunting. Fear is a signal. Be alert. Get vigilant. It wasn't that long ago that other humans or predators hunted us. This means you have to take action. You can't just sit and meditate your problems away; many meditators become my students because their abuse or rage doesn't go away by meditation alone. It does teach you how to get steady though. So get steady and now go out hunting.

Stalk your fears the way you'd stalk an animal. You might start out no-ticing a scuffle in the dirt that you recognize as a track, a little nibble and rub marks on the trees, a tiny tuft of fur that has rubbed off on a bush, a little pile of scat. These are all signs. When you get close enough, you'll smell the musk of the deer or hear that funny way they thump the earth with their hooves to make you back off. Fear will do the same thing—as you get closer, it'll do something to make you back off, to scare the hell out of you. Whatever it takes to make your heart pound, to get that stinky fear-sweat, to pump the adrenaline, or to sense that nasty taste in your mouth—those are all signs that you're getting close. Every time you hit a fresh pocket of terror, that's a useful sign; it'll take you to whatever most needs your attention. This takes courage! Keep going until you be-gin to close in on what's generating the fear. In the process, you'll make tremendous discoveries about yourself—an incredible treasure.

Sometimes our fears are based on past experiences or on what hap-pened around those incidents. Don't discount the experience that's causing your present fear—but recognize that it's only one of the expe-riences available. Sometimes our fear is triggered by a resemblance to something that put the fear there in the first place, like having a love af-fair that ended really badly, so you tell yourself, *I can't love again because it'll just kill me.* That fear may be just one of your stories.

When you hunt fear inside yourself, you're not going in to kill. Some of the greatest hunters are photographers because they have to get close enough to get a picture. You have to be really stealthy or build a blind—it takes hours of patience. Then you get your insight; what's creating this trail?

When you get to the source of your fear, that's when the real work starts. Just because you see the deer doesn't mean you've got dinner or the perfect photo. You're just ready for the next step: now what?

Then comes the process of unwinding the insight. Ask yourself, *Where does this come from in my life?* Track back through time. You may need to ask more questions to pinpoint what's going on—and again, you need to work with a mental health professional to do deep work. You won't always get an answer—ta-da, there it is!—but frequently you'll dis-cover how a past experience has archived your fear.

I was in northern California in the late seventies, careening along a mountain road, a snaky path along a cliff. I was showing off my 914 Porsche to a soon-to-be lover, being bold and adventurous and reckless. Suddenly I hit a slick patch, spun out, and cracked the car smack into the mountain, mere feet from a plunge off the cliff. I really banged up the car and myself and my friend—minor trauma but high drama. In an instant all that high reckless exuberant energy curdled into fear, shame, guilt—I'd endangered this man because I'd been so stupid. I became morose.

Later that year, I found myself in the passenger seat with a man I had been living with. We were heading down another wet mountain road in the driving rain. My feet were stomping so hard on the imaginary brake on the passenger side that my whole body tightened with fear. *What's this about?* I wondered. Oh, sure: my car accident. Man. Wet road. Driving too fast. "Slow down," I told this man. "I'm really scared." But when I hunted that fear, I realized that it wasn't really about the car accident at all. It was more about the desire for that high, exuberant, reckless feeling I'd had in that other relationship, which had all been woven into the accident. It took me a number of hunting trips until I realized what was going on. I missed the *delight* in that other relationship—that excitement and exuberance—that was absent from this one. The huge gift for persisting in the hunt was that when I realized I'd lost my exuberance for life, I got it back.

STOP MAKING DECISIONS BASED ON FEAR

Once you've located your fear, take a look at how it's made your life smaller. How does acting out of fear hurt you? When you figure that out, you're more open to making different choices. For example, I've worked with many women who stay in self-negating relationships because they're afraid to be on their own financially. They become what I call a Sacrificial Whore—someone who gives too much and who gets off on giving too much, whose reward for giving is to drain her own marrow. These women sabotage opportunities for richer relationships because they're afraid to strike out on their own.

Usually our fear comes from triggers that developed in an earlier, unpleasant situation. I have an aspect inside myself I call Firefighter— all of her triggers were developed during intense, terrible situations.

When I'm in a present situation that's intense but not terrible—perhaps I'm having an argument with a friend or I'm worried about someone's health—Firefighter comes up, flooding me with fear or rage or some other urgent feeling. When I respond from that fearful or panicky place, 99 percent of the time, I end up making terrible decisions.

Walking the Brave-Hearted Path means vowing to stop making decisions based on fear. To work with what I call a Warrior's Heart is to plant your feet when you feel that energy coming up, take a moment to sort through the signals you're sending yourself, and ask, *What is the most healing response that will bring me to a resolution I can be proud of?* When I act out of fear, I lash out. I'm most bewildered when I'm dealing with people I deeply, deeply love; I get swept away by the feeling and forget there's a path to be walked here. On the other hand, I don't want to kill Firefighter or lock her in a fireproof room; I want her to develop steadiness and discernment. I know the alarm bells are ringing; what's the most healing, helpful action, especially in a hot situation like an argument? To create a healing solution, make your decisions and good judgments based on your wise assessment after checking in with head, heart, gut, and pelvis—your chakras, wisdom and information centers that correspond to your endocrine system.

Some of us hide our fears behind noble causes, so we don't see how they hold us back. I had a client who was a banker. Her deep, passionate desire was to be a painter, but she chose this safe job to support her family and to avoid the angst of being the starving artist. I put her in Camel pose for a while. This was a radically uncomfortable position for her, and it brought up a lot of fears: *I can't do this. I'm afraid.* It was a very long time before she could say her heart's desire, "I want to be a painter." First she gave me all these reasons why she couldn't. I wasn't buying it. "Draw or paint me a picture by next week, and don't you dare cancel." She gave me a really good, detailed picture. It was the first time she'd drawn anything since she'd stepped away from art.

The act of drawing it had brought up painful and dramatic realizations. She discovered that she had turned from her heart and Spirit's desire. Finally she asked herself, *What if, once a week, I go into the laundry room and paint for twenty minutes?* She started taking art classes on family vacations, thus honoring her family as well as her needs as an artist. She'd have little breakthroughs, but then her old programming would take over and she'd get sick. But the more she reconciled the fear, the healthier she got and the more her Spirit returned.

FIND THE HEALING WITHIN THE FEAR

Once you've faced your dragon, your next task is to ally with it. Don't kill the beast, you fool, because that's your power! This is the archetypal hero's quest: You'll meet the dragons and the demons and fight and fight and fight them until you finally get the treasure. Then you'll depart that quest irrevocably changed, with that treasure a part of you. Every time you stalk your fear and choose life instead of oblivion, you'll begin to re-claim the parts of you that have been blocked off.

When you finally do get to that point of the fear's origin—*I'm still grieving the loss of that dream or hope; I'm still afraid because of that ac-cident*—you can make a Warrior's Choice to take a healing step at that very moment. That healing step might be very small; you might decide simply to take one deep breath, or not to numb yourself out with that slice of cheesecake, or to book a massage instead of doing a punishing hour at the gym, or to take a nap because your body is crying for sleep. But each small step takes you closer to your goal of healing.

The hero's choice is to disobey the dictates of the fear. Your fear may tell you to run, but don't do it. You can hit the wall of fear twenty-five times. It doesn't mean you failed if you ran away twenty-four times—if you've faced it once, you've succeeded.

I used to have recurring nightmares. When I'm in the midst of a re-ally big life-altering change, I'll frequently dream of T. rex. What could be more terrifying than something that fast, that big, with that many teeth? The T. rex would rampage through a little village (I have no prob-lem mixing my time periods) so fast, you could barely track it, snap-ping heads off, bearing off hapless humans. Sometimes I'd be running away, other times looking down on the carnage and feeling sad that I couldn't help my villagers. I'd wake up and write down every detail of my dream—the shame, the guilt. Writing it down started to break that conditioning that translated into my waking life: I'd get afraid, and then I'd choose not to act, wallowing in shame or guilt instead. But my dreams wanted me to make a better choice.

Then I started having a different kind of T. rex dream. It was stomping through the trees after me when suddenly I got really grounded and steady and shouted, "Wait!" T. rex stopped. That was weird. Then T. rex started to advance again. "No, wait!" I ordered it. T. rex stopped. Then I started playing with T. rex, walking under its legs, tickling its belly and balls (my humor has its own weirdness). I allied myself with this dragon. The terror was still huge, but I could still figure out how to join up with T. rex. All those legends say, "Kill the dragon," but the dragons were the ones who spoke the first words, the keepers of the oldest magic, the ones with the longest memories—why would you kill them just because they're more powerful and bigger than you? You can have a different response. Did I ever tame T. rex? No, but I began to build a strange alliance with it.

So how do you ally with your fear? How do you face the monster and tickle its belly? Because of my past, one of my greatest fears was of being a cripple. The solution turned out to be right in front of me. My fear was telling me, *If I'm crippled, I should die. I'd be worthless.* Then I got to thinking, *I've got a really good mind—it's good at problem solving.* What else could I do and still be a worthwhile human being who helps others? My first healing step was to find the answer to that question.

I started studying to be a therapist. You can be a healer without legs. My fear shifted radically because I found something else I could do that was extremely rewarding—energy work, hands-on stuff. I found the skills of therapy utterly fascinating. Yoga has its *asanas,* or poses and so does the psyche; therapy taught me those asanas as well. I started finding out how to work with things that had previously puzzled me—like how when I left people in poses for a long time, they would burst into tears. That's where the root of the healing was. In my work with horses, I had already perceived that hurtful experiences stored in muscle tissue could resurface. If a horse has been badly injured and frightened while jumping a certain kind of fence, it'll start limping when it sees that same particular jump, rolling his eyes, throwing his head back. Horses are so smart that they can create their own neuroses. (Sound familiar?)

I was terrified of becoming obese or a cripple, but my greatest fear was that I'd become just like my mother: a monster. Becoming a healer was a revolutionary way of using those fears. A fear journal teaches you to study your fear instead of run like hell from it, which is our natural inclination. I could become a catalyst for the release of people's fears from their bodies, but first I had to deal with my own. The therapist with whom I apprenticed was obese—crippled in his own way. He was also brilliant, with the talent, skill, and willingness to work with me and pull me through the abuse. Because of his care and skill, I was able to look beyond my initial disgust and revulsion regarding his obesity—the negative conditioning that had sprung from my relationship with my mother. My fear began to lose some of its claw-hold on me. That freed me to teach in a bolder and more compassionate way.

I learned how to go inside, feel the habitual internal response to something that scared me—and then hold steady and look for what else was inside. Then I had to come up with a creative solution that made me feel worthwhile and I could fascinate upon.

When you come up with a solution for allying—interacting and strategizing—with your fear, give yourself a decent trial period to see if it works. Can you fascinate upon this fear and honor that it had a purpose at one time?

SNUGGLE UP TO YOUR FEAR

I recommend you keep a fear journal as a way to snuggle up to your fear. A journal helps you give your fear a voice; you let it talk until it empties itself out. A fear journal teaches you to study your fear, which is radically different from our natural inclination, which is to run like hell from it. Write down each time you hit a fear, large or small. When did it come up? What triggered it? What did you feel? How did you respond? What healing step did you take? What solution might work better? The more you write down your fears and start tracking them, the more you'll zero in on what works and what doesn't.

How often is your fear twisting your response to your life? Keeping a journal helps you achieve clarity on your fear and avoid selective memories. Sometimes I don't recognize my own fear at first, but when I write down the actual sensations I notice—metallic taste, smelly sweat, clammy palms—I am able to say, "Oh, that's fear." The next time it gets triggered, I'll have a resource to access how I feel. My fear has gotten sneaky; it makes me forget what releases it. Writing it down makes it really obvious—Oh, when this person said these words, I went all numb because I got afraid and angry. So I stopped, took a few deep breaths, and then I was able to respond from a place of truth instead.

Some people's fears are more obvious. Let's imagine you come to one of my classes and tell me, "I'm afraid to go into Handstand because I could fall and snap my spine." That's a scary thought—there's truth to it. Then another scary thing happens: someone offers you help or you have to ask for help. Suppose you accept the teacher's help and she braces herself for any kind of fear dance you do—arms buckling, legs turning to water—so that no matter what, she's got you, you'll get to experience Handstand. That's a win. You'll have a whole different feeling in your body, a completely different chemical response. At the end of class, take out your journal and write it all down—how hard it was to ask for help or accept help. Every little detail you could track. Maybe you felt a glimmer of hope. What happened internally? What happened externally? Did you kick up a foot and then clunk back down? When you came down, what shifted? What's the win? Sometimes the win won't be a full-on chemical release or a huge epiphany, but it'll be *I did this, and I didn't get hurt* or *I did this, and I asked for help, and it was a trustworthy person, and I didn't get hurt* or *I asked a neighbor to spot me, and she was small, not strong, and didn't know how to help, and that was a mistake.*

Whether it's pushing yourself at Yoga or facing a fear at your job, on a date, at a party, or in your marriage, when you start writing things down in your fear journal, you start to see the wins.

Studying your fear changes your relationship to it and begins the exciting, terrifying breakthrough to freedom.

PHYSICAL FOCUS:
YOGA POSES TO ACCESS, PROCESS, AND RELEASE FEAR

Fear has a primal purpose to protect us. It lives in our cell tissue and tells us when to run, fight, or freeze. It's our job to learn to use it.

Our emotions leave chemical trails, and out-of-control fear exudes chemicals that make it easy for other hunters to find us. Fear has a very particular smell. Most animals can smell it, and so can I. Our ancestors burned up those stress chemicals in fight-or-flight reactions, but today we're in a perpetual freeze, never fully releasing the chemicals. Fear takes a powerful toll on our lives. The chemical processes triggered by fear can leave physical and emotional residues, which can lead to chronic health problems and, unexamined, even bizarre behavioral patterns like post-traumatic stress disorder.

When you're in that long-term pattern of fear-based response, it's like flooding poison throughout your system. There's nothing wrong with the adrenaline, but when it keeps happening without an outlet, it works like battery acid in the body. Learning a better way takes a while, but ultimately here's your choice: live with the fear and the health problems it creates, or go hunting. Which sounds tastier to you? Take courage. Hunt what makes you sick or sad or insane or terrified, so you can work free of the crippling fear.

Certain Yoga poses help access, process, and release fear. Inversions—upside-down poses—for example, are particularly useful. When people get into a pose and tell me, "I'm afraid of this," I say, "Awesome. Now I get to work with you in a safe way." I call it a fearasana. For some people it's Camel or Pigeon pose. Even Lunges, which prompt intense thigh action, will tap in to people's deep-seated emotions. The key is to work with the fear in the pose. Use the pose to stalk and hunt and entice your fear to come up so you can flush it free from your cell tissue. Then, when you come out of the pose, you can take that power and create your own personal tsunami, really jump in with both feet and bust through that situation that had you stuck, paralyzed with fear.

FOUR BASICS OF FORREST YOGA

Before I describe specific fear-busting poses, however, I want to introduce you to four basics of Forrest Yoga: deep breathing, tracking through feeling, active feet and hands, and a relaxed neck. When you walk into a Forrest Yoga class, you'll see immediately that the way we work with these basics differs from the typical Yoga class. Training yourself to work in this new way both on and off the mat will work wonders when you find yourself gripped or paralyzed by fear.

Deep Breathing

Breathing—it sounds too simple, so automatic. But in fact, when we're afraid, we hold our breath. We literally gasp for air. When we're in fear, we're not clearheaded or centered. Deep breathing will change your physiological response to fear, bringing fresh oxygen to every cell. You'll be able to think more clearly and assess situations without being frozen, blinded, or deafened by fear. Breathing correctly helps you move out pain, sparkles you up, and gives you better thinking power. Sound enticing? You just have to change the most automatic habit in your life— your breathing.

I learned to breathe by accident when I was a teenager. I'd come to visit a friend at a wildlife rehab center, and she greeted me accompanied by a wolf on a leash. I was really scared of that wolf. It was huge, with a completely feral look in its eyes that asked, *Are you lunch?* One look and I just stopped breathing, overcome with fear. Then I wandered around and came across a really big cage with a tiger in it. I'd never seen a live tiger, although I'd dreamed about them since I could remember. I hung out with this tiger for a really long time. And then I did a really stupid thing. I sidled up to that cage and started to pet this tiger. Soon I was scratching underneath this tiger's chin and throat, and he took his big soup pot head and kept pressing into my hand until it was flattened on the floor, his eyes were closing and his ears were twitching a little and his tiger teeth were hanging out the side. He was purring. I'd read that the big cats don't purr. I was watching this tiger and every tail twitch and flex of its claws inside its gigantic velvet paws. When this cat breathed, its whole ribcage expanded sideways and came back in. For some brilliant, unknown reason, I started breathing like that tiger—when I had my dreams of power, I *was* a tiger. It was amazing. My fear disappeared; I was flooded with energy. This big cat taught me how to breathe properly, so now I can teach you.

Begin by standing up straight, feet parallel and hip distance. Now tuck your tailbone down. Have you ever noticed that when you're afraid, you can't feel your pelvis? Tucking your tailbone turns on your buttocks muscles, which activates the pelvis and lengthens the spine, so you have better circulation of the cerebrospinal fluid, which gives you more energy and helps seat you into your root power. Our first two chakras, or energy centers—the flames of our life force—are right down in the pelvis.

Now pull in the low belly muscles from the navel on down. These are sleepier; they're supposed to be supporting the lower back, but they don't, so we have to teach them how. Activating these lower abdominal muscles also tones and stimulates the intestines.

Now inhale deeply, expanding your ribs sideways. On the exhale, pull the belly in and move the entire pelvic bowl in so that the tailbone reaches toward your heels and your buttocks muscles help pull the pelvic bones into this new position. Yes, you have to learn to use your ass to pull your tailbone down, which decompresses the back. Since we are a furniture culture, we have a lot of compression there, especially in the lower back, which leads to back pain, sciatica, dullness, and a lack of vital function in the intestines.

Tucking your tailbone and pulling your belly in when you're in fear helps break the fear up by forcing the energy to move through in a different way. It also taps the power of your buttocks muscles and legs.

Next telescope the ribs. In other words, lift your ribs away from your waist, lower back, and diaphragm, giving that area more space, which means you'll be able to take deeper breaths, which helps endurance and energy levels.

Now work on expanding the ribs. The easiest way to learn to do this is to put your hands on either side of your rib cage, exhale everything out, and feel how the ribs move in toward each other. Now, slowly, consciously inhale through your nose, feeling for how your ribs push against your hands as they expand. Instead of breathing down into your belly or up into your chest—breathe *outward*—feel the expansion of your ribs on the inhale and the contraction on the exhale. Feel for getting as many of the ribs to spread out as possible.

It takes a lot of practice to stay conscious and aware of your breathing. Later I'll teach you how to deepen that practice with Ujjayi breathing.

Tracking Through Feelings

We've gone pretty numb in our bodies. We've become very hard-working thinkers, but we've lost the wisdom available through the rest of our bodies, thus cutting off most of our chakras, our information centers. To restore that wisdom, we need to use our brains in a higher way. Thinking isn't the only gear we have. We also have feeling, which is a signal that tells us something; we need to learn how to make sense of the sensation in our bodies.

How do you track through feeling? There are two main components: visceral and emotional. The vehicle is the wind horse, your breath. Pigeon (see page 31 for an example of Pigeon pose) is a great pose to learn this in. In Pigeon we usually feel tight through our hips and legs. To track through feeling there, start by breathing into your lower back. Inhale and balloon your breath into your lower back so those back muscles expand outward. Even the littlest bit of movement means you're on the right track. Relax on the exhale.

Give yourself a few breaths in the pose to strengthen your connection to feeling. Now, inhaling, reach down with your deep breath, reaching toward the area where you're feeling the stretch. Hold your breath a moment, tighten your buttocks and leg muscles, then exhale and release those muscles. Now tighten those muscles again and release. Feel that? That's what the visceral sensation of release feels like. Stay connected to the sensation of your breath, moving your lower back and feeling the part of you being stretched in the pose. Inhale, bearing down so the breath reaches past the lower back into the pelvis. Hold your breath, tighten your pelvic muscles, exhale, and let go. Consciously relax around the tight spots as you exhale.

Keep doing this breath pattern. Be alert to how the sensation begins to ripple and change. This is where the emotional component might come in. Breathe down deeply as you let the waves of emotion come up and through you. An emotional release might show up as trembling, fear, tears, anger, or a desire to get up and bolt. Be curious about what's in that part of you. As the visceral sensation fluctuates, stay steady. Keep connecting to the visceral as well as the emotional feeling. Don't run away. Give yourself permission to feel the emotion. Keep breathing into the stretch, relaxing layer by layer with each exhale. Be brave enough to feel what's stuck in there and let it move. This frees up that part of your body. That new freedom is awesome.

Active Feet and Hands

When you walk into a Forrest Yoga class, one of the first things you'll notice is that participants use active feet and hands. They spread more weight throughout the whole foot by putting as much of the ball of the foot and the whole heel firmly on the ground as they can, then lifting their toes as far as possible off the ground and spreading them.

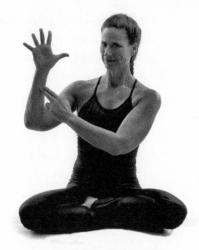

Active Hands and Feet

When we get fearful, we get caught up in our chest, neck, and jaw. Keeping your feet active makes the energy travel down to some of your biggest bones and muscles and makes you grounded, rooted. It also keeps you more aware because you're breaking a habitual posture. When your feet are active, you can't space out—it takes conscious volition to keep them that way. It won't ever be an automatic move, so you'll never go dull.

Active feet are as important off the mat as on. Keeping feet active is especially important if you sit at a desk, which can make it difficult to keep balance across your feet. Women, especially those accustomed to wearing high heels, may have more trouble with active feet at first because high heels scrunch the toes and keep the body off-balance, with the weight thrown forward. This makes the ankles unstable, which adds tension to the calves, butt, and back—and then into the upper back and neck. It's an unstable, fearful body position. Active feet can also help relieve pain from plantar fasciitis, an often intractable condition.

When you choose to work with active feet, you begin to feel how you walk through your life. Bringing that level of awareness into the steps you're taking has incredible consequences. When you're literally walking through a change—which is usually a most awkward time—you have a chance to walk with more integrity, grace, and in a way you can become proud of. You become a better problem solver instead of adding to the problem.

Make that desire to stay aware really tasty so you can evolve. Evolution is the best game in town, and there is no better high than an epiphany.

We use our hands to reach out to people or to push them away. Our hands are intimately connected to our heart, so when we get them active, there are direct and wonderful consequences for the heart. This is especially true if we are aware that reaching out with our hands means we're also reaching out with our hearts. If you reach for the keyboard, you want to make what comes out matter. Become more aware of how your hands move through your space, your life—what are they picking up? Frequently our hands will tell us if we're recoiling from something—they curl in, they get arthritic or cold and achy—all the signs of poor circulation. We're literally not moving energy through them. That's why we need active hands.

Put your hands palm down on the floor or a mat. Start spreading the bones of the heel of the hand as much as you can. Pull the skin and muscles across the palm taut. Spread all the fingers, moving the thumb and little finger as far away from each other as possible. Picture five lines of energy radiating out of your fingertips, as if they could emit light. Now reach the finger bones away from the wrist. This brings space and strength to the bones, ligaments, tendons, and muscles of the hand and wrist. Make sure the middle finger faces forward. Apply pressure through the web of skin between your thumb and forefinger. When you press down onto your hands, be careful not to rest all the weight on the heel of the hand. Press more through the top of the palm where the fingers meet; that helps lengthen the wrist. Push back so the energy and weight of the arm and body doesn't fall into the wrist. It's as though you were walking on your hands, pushing as though you were stepping.

Keeping your hands active helps to relieve compression in the wrist and hand bones as occurs in carpal tunnel syndrome or from any gripping action. I work with a lot of professional golfers who put a death grip on those clubs. Baseball players, computer wizards cupping around the mouse, cooks gripping tools—we all grab so hard that we damage our hands; keeping them active eases much of the pain while also teaching us a lighter grip.

Relax the Neck

Relaxing the neck is essential for changing
your response to fear. Stand up straight,
get your feet active, take a deep breath,
and expand your ribs. Exhale. Now move
your right ear toward your right shoulder, but keep your shoulder down. Don't
push the head—*relax* it. All you intensity
junkies and type-A personalities, please
reread this line: *relax the neck; don't push
it.* Feel the stretch on the left side of your
neck. Breathe into the stretch, feeling for
relaxing the neck a little more with each
breath. Do this for three to five breaths.

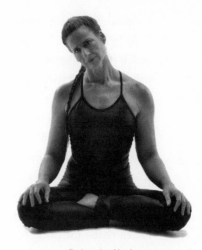

Relax the Neck

Then, cradling the right side of the head with the right palm, use the
hand to bring your head upright to center. Yes, I know you can use your
neck to lift your head—*but don't.* Now do the other side.

Those of us who live high-stress lives experience a perpetually tight
neck and jaw, which sends fear signals throughout the body that create
a constant level of anxiety, which our body reads as fear. This constant
fear leads to adrenal stress, exhaustion, irritability, cloudy thinking, delicate or upset stomach, constipation, or the runs. Relaxing the neck helps
release the claw-grip of fear and sends a signal of relief and relaxation to
the nervous system. The intelligence of your brain can now communicate with the wisdom of the rest of your body. The brain is nourished by
oxygen and cerebrospinal fluid, which means that a relaxed neck allows
us to make better decisions and stop reacting out of sluggishness and
anxiety and confusion.

PREPARING FOR THE POSES

Once you've learned these four basics of Forrest Yoga, you're ready to
use some specific poses to help address and release fear. This takes time
and patience. Just going into a pose, feeling a pull, and moving out of it
doesn't give it time to build, marinate, and release. Give it a little foreplay,
a little time. Stay in the Yoga pose because that's like shining a light on

the trail of your fear. If you come out of it right away, you may get a flash of insight or intuition, but more likely the feeling will subside and you'll be left with, "That was awful—I'm never doing that again," when in fact you just needed to follow it through. Give the muscles time to release.

Next step: be willing to breathe and feel and let the cell tissue get stimulated enough that the old, stuck stuff can drain out. Five deep breaths aren't enough, even if they're sweet. Take ten breaths minimum. Track the sensation; if you sense a rush of heat or feel like you want to scream, break down, or cry, all of that is a sign of release. Let's say you're in Bridge pose. Your butt's up in the air, your legs are trembling, your crotch is shoved up toward the ceiling. That pose could begin to tap in to cell tissue memory. A lot of fear comes up when we tap deeply in to the thighs. Notice how when you're really scared, your legs turn to water? We don't have a physical outlet for that chemical response to fear. So when we do Bridge pose, around the tenth breath, the position begins to stimulate the area that the particular experience is layered into. It's very peculiar—here you are on your Yoga mat and suddenly you're scared spitless. It makes no sense at all until you're skilled in this form of tracking. Stay with it.

You might feel as if lava is moving through your thighs, down your shins, through your feet. When that burning starts, it's scary and intense. Recognize: This is not a bad thing, not an injury about to happen. It's about a cleansing of the past from your cell tissue. Be willing to let that swell of feeling build so you can ride that wave. Sometimes you'll begin the ride and you have to get off—it's too intense. That's okay; you rode it for a few seconds. That's honorable. Next time you might ride it for four seconds. When that fear or rage or feeling comes up, you're on the right track. Give it a few more breaths. Can you negotiate with your fear a little bit? Can you take two more breaths, staying really present? Your goal is to get past the struggle and thrash.

When we struggle, we become our most stupid self. We lose contact with our deep breath, we forget all of our resources, we move in a desperate, injuring way, and then we quit—none of which is helpful for progression. If your backside is burning, that's okay, that's not an injury—that's energy getting ready to release. Sometimes it's rage. When our power has been stopped or shut down, we can feel rage at having our boundaries crossed and our creativity thwarted. This anger can get stopped up in the thighs and pelvis. For the love of the people you care about, ride those waves of intensity until they crest and break—breathe and release it before you leave the mat. If it took you ten breaths to reach that peak of intensity, it may take another ten breaths to release it. That's time well spent.

Keep tracking the emotional backlog through the pose. This will eventually lead you to the story of your own life, in which you made a crucial series of decisions that affect you forever because of the backlog still sitting in your cell tissue. With each tracked emotion, you clean a little layer out, but you also explore your own fear edge. You're tracking something that's exciting because it changed your life—you just don't know how until you've tracked it all the way. You begin to question the decisions you made back then. You can choose to live differently now.

LUNGE

When you move into Lunge, you're dealing with big muscles—quadriceps—so it takes a while for the pose to take its effect. This pose is so

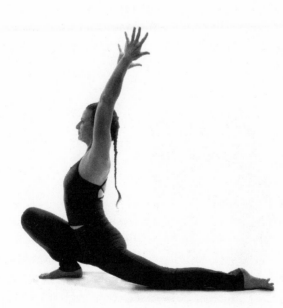

Lunge

simple, and it works deeply. Anatomically, it's straightforward, but energetically and physiologically, it's a mover and a shaker.

Inhale and step your left leg back into a lunge. Sink your hips toward your front heel, bending the right knee deeply. Keep your front heel flat and lift your ribs and arms, keeping your hands and feet active. Spread the fingers and tuck your tailbone. Take ten deep breaths; then switch to the other side. Notice the vitality in your legs and pelvis, which feels really good. It's much easier to connect to your power once you've done lunges because it unlocks those barriers to that vitality.

If you have knee pain, adjust the pose. If the front knee is bothering you, be sure the ankle is aligned under the knee. If the back knee is bothering you, put layers of padding under it.

CAMEL

Camel is a good pose for cleansing the toxic residue of fear. When we're afraid, we close down in our chest and shield our heart, but Camel begins to melt those shields. It also strengthens the back, stretches out the belly, and opens the front of the pelvis.

To warm up properly for Camel, do eight Sun Salutations (see page 223) first. Kneel with your knees and feet two to four inches apart. Tuck your tailbone down and telescope your ribs up to keep the compression out of your lower back. Keep your chin down toward your chest. Place your hands on your sacrum, thumbs by your spine, fingers pointing to-

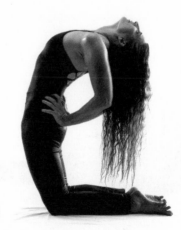

Camel

ward your hips. Breathe in, puffing up your chest. Lift your heart while using the buttocks muscles to tuck your tailbone down. If you don't have any neck problems, a different head position is to relax your head back and open the throat—a very vulnerable position. Press down through the shins to help you telescope your ribs, moving the energy right out through the heart. Ride the intensity. Take ten breaths. The longer you stay in the pose, the richer the return.

If you feel any back pain, make sure your tailbone is tucked and your ribs telescoped, lifting away from your lower back. Camel is a real thigh burner. Pain in the front of the thighs is okay, but if you feel any pain in the knees, separate them a bit more.

To transition out of the pose, straighten your torso, then sit down on your heels, put your hands on your lower back, and breathe into the lower back.

PIGEON

Pigeon is a great soother of the nervous system. If you've had something really scary happen to you—perhaps you had a scary fall—Pigeon flushes out the fear like rainwater. Since it releases and opens the hips, sacrum, and lower back, Pigeon is great for sciatica and tight hamstrings. Pigeon releases stress at the end of the day, so it's a nice pose to do before bed once you're comfortable with it; it'll help you relax, open, unwind.

Start by sitting with your left leg forward, your left foot close to your right hip and your right leg straight behind you. (As you become more advanced, you can move that shin closer to parallel with the front of the mat.) Lean over your front shin, keeping your hips level. Beginners

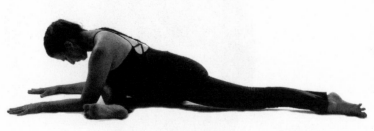

Pigeon

can put their forearms on the floor with elbows beneath their shoulders; more advanced folks can lay their torsos down onto the front leg. Pull your shoulders away from your ears. Keeping your feet active, reach through the back leg. Breathe into the low back and left hip. Hold the pose for ten breaths, and then repeat on the other side.

Since you're working with very big pelvic and thigh bones, opening them can give you quite a sweet rush, which can be pretty exciting if you've got a lot locked up there. However, that big release of energy can be scary. If an emotional wave comes up—fear, anger, whatever—keep breathing and ride it. As the intensity increases, deepen your breath to meet it, which will help the wave swell and crest and break. If you ride the wave until it breaks, the release is a relief; relaxation will wash through you, and you'll sleep really sweetly.

DOWN DOG ON THE WALL

Down Dog and Down Dog on the Wall are important steps in working up to holding Handstand. They help your body get used to being upside down. When you can hold Down Dog for eight breaths, move on to Down Dog on the Wall. When you can hold that for ten breaths, it's time to try Handstand.

To do Down Dog, get down on your hands and knees, facing away from the wall, with your feet about twelve inches from it. Curl your toes

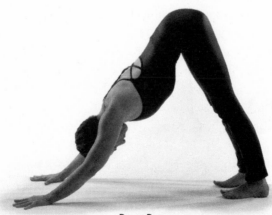

Down Dog

under, straighten your knees so your feet move back, and move into an upside-down vee with your heels touching the wall. Press your chest toward your legs.

To move into Down Dog on the Wall, inhale and step one leg at a time three feet up the wall. Your legs should be parallel to the floor and your torso perpendicular to it. Work up to holding this for ten breaths, and then step down one leg at a time directly to the floor.

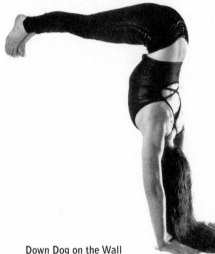

Down Dog on the Wall

HANDSTAND

A lot of people are really scared of being upside down; it can bring up a lot of stuff. My theory is that this stems from the way most of us traditionally enter the world: we're born, freezing, wet, upside down, strafed by piercing bright lights—and then we get hit until we cry! I remember working with my friend Janos, who was 6'2" and about two hundred pounds of scared person—fear is heavy!—to help him overcome his terror of Handstand. When he got it, he was able to grapple with the other fears in his life.

Handstand is exhilarating. As it activates your endorphins, it uplifts and washes your energy clean in a minute. Your eyes will perceive things differently because you've just washed the film off them and rinsed,

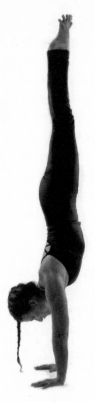

Handstand

refreshed, and activated your brain. Handstand sweeps away negative and obsessive thinking; you simply can't obsess while you're in this pose—you'll fall right out. This pose is so much better for lifting depression and low energy than coffee is—and without the extreme mood swings. So if you need a lift, go for this pose instead of a cup of coffee, a cigarette, a glass of wine, or Coke (either kind). It's also great for the guts, since it reverses the pull of gravity on your internal organs. It builds strength in your arms, legs, chest, and upper back. It's also great for building self-esteem; when you come down, you'll feel strong, having met the challenge. The achievement of balance, even for a moment, is a revelation. Staying up for a while takes a lot of practice. That we can balance so exquisitely, even in this moment of intensity, is a great life teaching . . . and what a victory when you get it!

Avoid Handstand if you have wrist or shoulder injuries or a detached retina. If you're pregnant or have osteoporosis, check with your Yoga teacher and health care professional. If you get the go-ahead, your Yoga teacher must spot you going into *and coming out of* the pose.

Handstand requires some preparation; you don't just want to fling yourself into it without any warm-up. To prepare for Handstand, I recommend six Elbow to Knee (see page 58), six to twelve Sun Salutations (see page 223), and then either Down Dog for eight breaths or Down Dog on the Wall (see page 33) for five to ten breaths.

To begin, start with a wall well away from any windows and clear all the space around you so you don't land on anything. Women, this is a good practice. Learn to move obstacles out of your way instead of moving yourself around the obstacles!

Practice kicking up to the wall. Physiologically it's easier to start from standing, but psychologically, it's easier to get up into a handstand if you start with your hands on the ground. This is where the fearasana comes in; it can be scary to go upside down. Ideally, you'll have a spotter, but we don't always have people around to keep us precisely safe, so let the wall act as your safety net.

Plant your fingertips about six inches from the wall, fingers spread and facing the wall. Focus on your smart leg. (If you're right-handed, your right leg is probably your smart leg, and vice versa.) Point the smart toe back toward the floor about three or four inches behind the other foot. Inhale deeply. On the exhale, swing your smart leg up as strongly as possible, letting the other leg follow. (Be careful not to hold your breath; it'll make you stiff and weigh four hundred pounds.) Keep strong lines of energy through your arms so they don't buckle. Keep your legs as straight as possible once they're both up on the wall. Push against your hands, lift up out of your shoulders, and let your neck hang relaxed. Tuck your tailbone toward your heels, squeeze your inner thighs and ankles together, lift through the balls of your feet on the big toe side, spread your toes for balance, and breathe evenly. Focus your gaze on a spot on the floor to help you find balance. To cool down afterward, do a standing forward bend or Neck Release (see page 64).

If you don't get up the first hundred times, don't get frustrated; just enjoy the play of practice, including learning how to land lightly with integrity and balance instead of a big splat. Your challenge is to feel for how to stay connected all the way up and down as you move through unknown space and establish new neurological pathways. It's thrilling to track it!

Make the decision to track your fear, to turn from prey to predator. When you become the hunter, you create new opportunities for grace and growth. Once you choose to walk the Brave-Hearted Path, you can begin to let go of the old stories that have chained you to your past and move into an exciting unknown: the uncharted territory of your future.

2

WALKING FREE OF PAIN:
SUFFERING IS OPTIONAL

SNUGGLES WAS one devious mare, always getting loose from her stall, a real escape artist. One day she'd somehow gotten out again and was trotting around the big corral. Every time the other stable brats or I tried to grab her halter, she leaped away. No surprise there; Snuggles was a total bitch, even when she wasn't in heat. When she was in heat, she was really a drama queen. That day I'd had about enough of her antics. I ran up right behind her to try to grab her.

Wham! She fired right back at me with one of her hind legs, hitting me smack in the face. I could feel her metal shoe cutting my lip above my teeth and the force of her kick throwing me to the ground. The whole world slowed down as I just sat there, watching numbly as this drip drip drip of blood from the huge gash in my face pooled in the dirt in front of me. I gingerly poked my tongue through the new hole in my cheek. "Holy shit. You okay?" one of the stable kids wanted to know. For once I had no snappy comeback. Snuggles had kicked my usual snarky attitude right out of me.

I somehow picked myself up and limped down to Nick's office, wondering whether I'd broken anything.

"Jesus, what did you do to yourself?" He plunked me down on a stool, pulled my chin toward his old wrinkly face, and picked out the gravel, dirt, and horse manure from my cut. Now it hurt like hell. He washed off the blood, squeezed on some nasty-smelling purple liquid disinfectant, and packed the cut with Corona horse cream. "You're going to have a scar there," he told me, roughly but not unkindly. "Like a trophy. It'll be cool."

"She was running right behind Snuggles," one of the kids told him.

"That was stupid," Nick said, like I didn't know. He pointed to my cut. "It'll be something to remind you not to be stupid." By now my head was pounding and my eyes felt gritty from the dirt and holding back tears of pain and humiliation. "Come on, kid, get up," he told me. "Get over it."

I stumbled through my chores at the stable, fetching horses for folks going out on trail rides, grooming them, mucking out stalls. My face was numb, burning, and throbbing all at the same time, and my body hurt all over. A few hours later, there was Nick in the corral, jumping rope with the lead lines. "Hey, Annie, come join me!" I ached everywhere, but how do you refuse the invitation of a sixty-year-old man jumping rope? Pretty soon I was bouncing up and down right along with him. That was Nick's approach to pain—just deal with it and get moving.

It hadn't taken long for Nick's place, Azusa Canyon Stables, to become my real home. His was a rent stable—trail horses for hire, some boarders, and a few school horses that riders could train on for show. It was an impossible distance from my home—fifteen miles. So I learned how to hitchhike there within a year or two of discovering it.

Nick was a wild man, a short, bow-legged, wiry fellow with a big voice. He still had an eye for people living on the edge from his days working at a circus. At about six, I was the youngest by far of a ragtag bunch of stable brats—druggies and drinkers, smokers and dealers. Nick didn't care about our flaws. He took us all in, taught us how to care for the horses, how to take people out on trail rides. He was always barking at us like a terrier, but there was affection beneath his brusque demeanor.

In exchange for stable work, Nick also taught me how to ride. When I first got to his stables, my ankles were so weak, I could stand on the insides of them. My knees and back were always throbbing with pain.

Those corrective orthopedic shoes I was forced to wear were torture devices. Whenever I walked, I felt like the little mermaid from Hans Christian Andersen's story, each step grinding away like a dull knife blade. My legs were so weak that the first time Nick sat me on a horse—Sunny, a big fat palomino—I just slid right off his back the second he took a step. Nick laughed and told me to get on again. As I gradually found the ability to hold on, I began to think less about my bum legs; when I did, I'd think, *Who cares? I have four strong legs underneath me. Even better!*

All I knew is that I somehow had to keep moving to get away from the awfulness inside my parents' house. At first I would just run down the railroad tracks. I'd just head down those tracks as long as I could—until I fell down—to try to get the crazies out. Hours later I'd walk back to the house, step by painful step. Then I started disappearing for a few days. I didn't exactly know how to have friends, but I'd find some person who was willing to let me sleep at their house. Sometimes I'd find a bench I could sleep under. Before too long, I was spending nights at the stables. First I tried sleeping in the stalls, but I'd just get stepped on. So I'd sleep out in the cold, huddled in a haystack. I owned coats, but I could never seem to remember to bring them to the stables. I couldn't put it together how to care for myself—when I couldn't stand the cold or exhaustion anymore, I'd just curl up wherever I was and try to get some sleep. Nick didn't mind my hanging out all the time, and certainly my parents weren't going to come looking for me.

I was always getting run over, chomped, or kicked at the stables. Nick's attitude toward dealing with pain was always: *No big deal. Just patch me up and set me back on my feet.* I was still relying on my parents' liquor cabinet, sneaking out to it at night, taking tiny sips from the pretty bottles to ease the pain. It helped, especially when I woke up after what felt like blackouts, with my head feeling like it had been split in half. But the other stable brats had an edgier approach. Five or six years older than me, they preferred getting high and popping pills. Soon I was sharing their pills and weed too—anything to keep up with them, to feel like I belonged, and to stay numb. I was grateful for the whites—uppers—and NoDoz they gave me; I liked the go-go-go stuff that kept me awake because I hated the nightmares that continued to haunt me.

You can't be a runaway if no one's chasing you; I was more of a walk-away. Once my mother demanded, "Where were you?" I answered truthfully: "Doing drugs. Drinking. If you don't want to know, don't ask me." She pretty much stopped asking me after that.

As Nick took me more and more under his wing, he began teaching me how to doctor the horses. One day I was walking around the stables when I got the sense that something was wrong. I checked on the horses in the stalls first; they were all fine. So I went to the corral where we kept the rent horses. All of them were eating the hay we'd just put down except for Diamond Jim, a drooping gelding who stood off to the side by himself. He looked sick and sad, with a bulging lump on his throat. I went to get Nick. He took one look and told me that Diamond Jim had distemper and the lump was an abscess that was slowly choking off his breathing. "Here, Annie, you hold his head steady," Nick told me. I gripped Diamond Jim's halter and lead line, my toes barely skimming the ground. As Nick took a lance to the horse's abscess, Diamond Jim reared up, lifting me right off the ground. He threw his head back, and foul-smelling pus sprayed out all over my face and front, but still I held on tight. Nick roared with laughter, but I could tell he was impressed that I hadn't let go.

Nick said that Diamond Jim would probably die, but I decided to make him my personal project. His wound needed constant tending; it developed what's called proud flesh—thickened, scarred tissue that we had to carefully clean out again and again. This was a painful process for Diamond Jim—to get at the healthy tissue, we had to break down the proud flesh, cutting it away, cleaning it with caustic, peeling away the dead scabs. But it was a necessary step to get rid of the stuff that was diseased and dead so Diamond Jim could achieve true healing. Slowly, slowly, the light began to come back to Diamond Jim's eyes. He got better, and I began to feel that there was a healer within me.

In turn, over the years, the horses were starting to heal me. They were so big, beautiful, unpredictable; they represented freedom, power. On my own feet, I could walk and run, but it always hurt. On a horse, I was *big*, and I could go places. Riding was a different kind of pain, but if it took me somewhere, I was willing to put up with it. I *loved* riding, and the pain in my legs didn't matter because I'd never learned that pain mattered. My connection with the horses was the beginning of freedom, though I didn't quite know what that was. There was such a yearning inside me when I was around them; I just had to touch them.

This brought a revelation: there were ways they liked to be touched, and ways they didn't. I didn't know that there were all different kinds of touch. To me, touch was bad and loud and hurtful. But the horses liked hard scratching on their bellies, soft stroking on their noses, gentle itching on their ears—a whole array of feeling that could be evoked by where and how I touched. That blew my mind. It was like opening a door and finding a world made out of velvet. Horses spoke to a part of me that had never been touched or fed.

At the same time I was starting to develop a kind of feeling with the horses, almost a kind of love, I also had these moments of horror and great shame. Something ugly was beginning to bubble up inside me. Sometimes if I got stomped or bit—a not uncommon occurrence—I found myself flipping into a monster like my mother, kicking or striking the horse repeatedly. It was as if I'd been infected by my mother's wild sense of righteousness and brutishness.

It was just one more sign of how broken I felt. Here I was, at the beginning of discovering a sensation of openness, something beyond pain and numbness, and my curious delight was immediately tainted with shame whenever I went into those crazed rages. Why was I doing this? Would I become like my mother? And how would I get myself to stop?

The way out of some of my pain came from a challenge from someone I barely knew. When I was about thirteen, a girl named Robin Smith came up to me at school. "I have something you can't do," she told me.

Robin was a short kid, soft-spoken, very pale, and a little overweight. By now I was one hard kid, toughened up by all my work at the stables, feeling pretty strong. I looked her over and thought, *Sure, right.* I took out my cigarettes, tamped one down, lit it with my hand cupped around it in my best tough kid act, and barked, "Yeah, what?"

"Yoga. Want to go to class with me?"

To this day, I don't know what made that girl approach me and issue that challenge; we barely knew each other. I think it was a nudge from what Native Americans call the Sacred Ones. Robin took me to my first Yoga class. I was completely shocked. Here were all these ancient ladies—they were probably all of thirty years old—reaching forward and grabbing their toes, rolling onto their bellies into bow pose, backs arcing gracefully as they grasped their ankles. These were ordinary people, not circus folk, moving fluidly in and out of these beautiful poses. The best I could do was lean forward and grab behind my knees.

I started going to Yoga class regularly. Robin dropped out, but I was hooked. Shirley Pepping, my first teacher, was astonishingly gifted. Here was this mother with a beautiful body, red hair, china blue eyes— I thought, *How could she look like that and be so old?* She overthrew my paradigm of what I understood a mother to be. A mother could be more than merely someone who bore children and then grew hideously fat as she hissed about her progeny sucking her dry like parasites. Shirley drew me to my salvation and modeled for me a new way to be a woman.

The Yoga poses were painful and I was awful at them, but I kept going—life was painful, so what? The only part I couldn't stand was the end of class, when Shirley led us through Savasana, or Corpse pose. *You want me to lie down and relax with a bunch of people? Hell no!* Whenever I did, belly exposed, I just felt unbearably vulnerable. When Shirley tried to take us on a guided journey—"Now we're floating down a river . . . now we're riding on a cloud"—it'd be all I could do not to leap to my feet and scream, "Fuck you!" It all felt too familiar in an unpleasant way, too much like brainwashing. It would be years before I could lie down and relax, years before I understood why I felt so vulnerable lying in that position.

Slowly, my Yoga improved. One day I woke up and realized that something was missing: the pain in my legs and back. And while I couldn't yet deal with the emotional pain in my life, I began to understand that I was suffering emotionally. That itself was a huge step for me.

Through Yoga I saw that we humans have our own proud flesh. The body locks our traumas inside and archives them for future discovery and, hopefully, healing. Each trauma needs to be unraveled and eased, the scars opened, massaged, and broken down. The body can become like a tree that's root-bound and dying; the roots need to be very gently pulled apart, not just hacked off. That's the healing role of Yoga. And that's what began to happen for me.

THROUGH THE DOOR OF PAIN

There's a difference between good pain and bad pain. Like fear, pain is a red flag that means "proceed with caution"—pay attention, get interested—but it *doesn't* mean "go numb and stupid." It can be like a dark prison cell: you can put your head down and try to blast through the wall (the athlete's approach), you can back away from the wall and stay imprisoned (as many do), or you can reach out and really explore the wall until you find the door, open it, and step free. That's the path of Forrest Yoga.

There are three different types of pain—physical, emotional, and spiritual. It can be very difficult to tease these apart because they're often intertwined, and all types of pain show up physically; a broken heart might show up as clogged arteries, lung issues, and heart disease. Why it manifests a certain way is part of the mystery of each person's makeup and how that person operates from that deep wound.

For example, one of my students began working with me just after she'd had fallopian tube surgery following a failed pregnancy. Malka told me that she basically felt nothing below the waist. Yet she was a walking contradiction, telling me over and over, "No feeling; it hurts. No feeling; it hurts." She was in a paradoxical state of numbness *and* agony. My work with Malka consisted of helping her process through both emotional and physical pain together.

First I had Malka shut her eyes and do a special abdominal exercise called Agni Sara—Cleansing by Fire. Each time she pulled her stomach in, I had her pull her genitals up. I placed her hands on her abdomen and asked her to send breath there and feel those muscles push out against her fingertips. Gradually that pain began to dissipate and Malka began to realize that her emotional numbness had prevented her from dealing with a deeper issue: her grief about not having children. She'd lost one of her life's great desires—a huge part of her cultural conditioning had told her she was worthless if she couldn't have children, and her response had been to encapsulate her heart, pelvis, and belly around that numbness. Once she learned to work through the numbness, she not only helped herself walk free of pain, but she became much more charismatic, much braver. All from confronting her pain and working with her heart.

I'll show you how to break the habits that keep you in emotional, physical, and spiritual pain. The Formula for Change is a step-by-step primer for breaking those bad habits and embracing more healing actions. The Yoga poses can help you walk free of pain. I'm not saying that you'll never have pain, but you can change your relationship with it. You can rid yourself of the thoughts around pain that make you suffer. These tools and skills will help you move more adeptly through life's challenges and hurts. And then, if you experience a physical injury, you can learn how to heal it, which is very empowering.

SPIRITUAL FOCUS:
HEALING PAIN BEGINS WITH BREAKING UNHELPFUL PATTERNS

We are intensely habitual creatures, and many of our habits don't serve us. Most of us have pain because we've fallen into bad patterns: physical, emotional, and spiritual ones. To heal pain, we need to break those patterns, which can be surprisingly challenging. Don't believe me? Try this: clasp your hands. Look at which thumb and forefinger are on top. Now, interlace your fingers again with the *other* thumb and forefinger on top. That weird, awkward, uncomfortable feeling? It's called change. And it's *hard.*

Our minds run the same mazes as our bodies do. We think that when we decide to change, we should be able to do it instantly. Not so! We need to spend time breaking old patterns, then building and walking new neurological connections and pathways in order to make lasting changes.

The most important pattern to break and reset is how you breathe. When I ask my students: "What can't you live without?" they pepper me with the usual responses: "Oh, I can't live without love/spirit/kindness/chocolate/coffee/cocaine/my partner." Wanna bet? Sure you can. It might not be fun, might not be pleasant, but you'd soldier on. Here's what you can't live without: your breath.

We breathe all the time, and yet when we put our attention on something that automatic, we can begin to explore that vast internal wondrousness inside us. How great to find that grand expanse, that Great Mystery of the cosmos, inside our own skin!

No matter what the origin of your pain, learning to ride your own breath—your wind horse—will help take you through it. We're so habituated to struggle that it seems we just have to live with it, but breathing into our pain instead of thrashing around it opens the door to healing.

Arthur was a typical struggler. You could hear it in his breath, see it in his big muscles. He was a big believer in *No pain, no gain* and that whatever he was doing didn't count unless it came at a great cost—physical or emotional. Whatever pose he was in, he'd be doing his Mr. Macho grunting. One day while fighting and grunting in Bridge pose, he finally decided to release the struggle and just ride his breath into the pose. That breath's freedom cascaded into a realization that brought him to tears: his whole life was about struggle. The moment he just stopped struggling and moved into breath, that whole paradigm fell apart. That single, visceral epiphany changed a toxic habit that had brought enormous pain into his life.

Start feeling your breath. When you're stressed or angry or in pain, do you hold it? Do you pant and grunt and groan through struggle? Take four or five long, deep breaths. Feel how they energize you. Can you begin to change the habitual way you breathe, to reconnect with feeling your breath and then to deepen it, no matter what?

HOW TO BREAK A BAD HABIT: THE FORMULA FOR CHANGE

It takes a lot of commitment to break a bad habit, even one that's causing you pain. Make the decision now: Are you ready to change? If you want to succeed in breaking that toxic pattern and building a healthier pathway, be willing to take what I call a Soul Pledge—yeah, it's that serious!—to stay alert, conscious, aware. I've made and broken many commitments and resolutions to myself; when I make a Soul Pledge, however, that's an unbreakable vow to myself, one I will keep no matter what. You need to dig deep to hunt what's causing the pain on a physical, emotional, and spiritual level. Practice staying alert so you can stop obeying the external dictates that brought you to this painful state.

When you've taken that pledge, you're ready for the Formula for Change, a four-step tool I invented to help you banish a behavior that's bringing you pain so you can replace it with a healing action. In summary, here are the steps:

1 Catch that You're Doing the Behavior

2 Take Ten Deep Breaths and Reset

3 Reward Yourself Lavishly for Catching the Behavior

4 Take One Step Toward Healing

Let's go into detail on how to take each of these steps.

Catch that You're Doing the Behavior

Now, for the coming week, play detective to track any habits that exacerbate your physical pain or injuries. Get excited; you're on a mission. Start getting into a problem-solving frame of mind; in order to break a pattern, you first have to recognize it. Similarly, pay close attention to what makes your emotional pain worse. How does your body respond to it? How can you change it?

Some physical pain has a straightforward cause. Start by looking for an unconscious physical component; those are the easiest to spot. Are you sleeping in a way that puts a kink in your neck? Did you know your posture while you drive or sit at a computer can lead to headaches or migraines? Men tend to aggravate their back pain and sciatica by putting their wallet on the same side of their pants—so they sit in their car, chair at work, etc., on top of that wallet, which throws the hips and sacrum off. How do you sit at your computer? If you slump, you'll end up with a foggy brain, neck pain, an achy back, and pain radiating into your arms and hands through the brachial nerves.

Stay awake during those most boring, unconscious moments of your day—for example, how you turn your head when you change lanes in your car—because it's in those blanked-out moments that you can set yourself up for pain. Kinking your neck while changing lanes can stress the nerves and disks in the neck, especially if you're a tense driver.

Wanda had a shoulder injury. Her left shoulder would always improve when we did Yoga together, but days later, when she came back, she'd be in pain again. She was in a lot of despair. One day I walked Wanda out to her car after class and watched as she got in and went to fasten her seat belt. She reached with her left hand, palm facing forward, to fasten her seat belt in a way that was totally tweaking her shoulder—*that* was the move she needed to catch that was causing her trouble. I taught her how to reach over with her right hand and pull the seat belt across. Stopping that habit didn't heal that shoulder, but now Wanda could quit reinjuring it so the work we were doing could heal it. Her chronic pain began to fade.

Emotional pain can be harder to track. It can show up physically, but not necessarily in the part of the body where you think it should be. Dealing with someone who's a pain in the ass may not cause you a pain in your ass! But sometimes the body does speak literally. You may end up with heartburn because a conflict with someone is more serious than you've acknowledged—it hurts your heart. You might have a stiff, achy neck because of lousy posture—or because your neck muscles have tightened protectively because you're afraid to speak your truth.

If you've had intense surgery, that area may have been sensitized, so it can function as an early warning system. Pay attention—this area is talking to you. If something hurts and you can't uncover a physiological reason for it, ask: *What am I holding that I need to move through?* Treat pain as a barometer rather than a reason to go into victim mode. It's a signal; pay attention and address it. Go diving. Something like colitis might have been triggered by a habitual stress response to your SOB boss, drinking too much coffee (a common irritant that makes nerves more raw and reactive), not getting enough sleep, or any combination of causes.

How do you react to the challenges and stresses in your life? Feel where they affect your body, and get alert. Once you've identified the behavior that's causing or aggravating pain, watch for it, catch it, and then *stop*! Make a different choice instead.

Take Ten Deep Breaths and Reset

Your next step after catching your behavior is to take ten deep breaths. Then change your physical position. Our habitual behavior has a habitual posture, a habitual breathing pattern, and a habitual internal dialogue, so when you change your position, you change all of it. This will get your energy up and support you, and give you a quiet mind to ask: *What's the most healing step I can take at this time? See a doctor? Go into therapy? Take a Yoga class?* Taking those breaths and changing your position will make a difference in how you walk through life.

Reward Yourself Lavishly for Catching the Behavior

Let's say you catch yourself falling into that bad habit that causes pain. Maybe you're still slumping at your computer, causing yourself physical pain. Or you're thinking self-mutilating thoughts like *My belly is so flabby; I'm so ugly,* causing emotional pain. Stop and take a few deep breaths to re-center yourself. The temptation is to beat yourself up when you catch yourself doing the same damn thing again—*I'm such an idiot! Why do I always do this to myself? Why can't I learn?* But that'll just dig that well-worn groove even deeper and lead to shutdown and numbness, making you more dull and less effective. *Do not punish yourself.* It takes some discipline not to go into that abrasive internal monologue because we think that if we self-mutilate, we're being good disciplinarians, but it doesn't work. I'm not saying that any indulgent, aberrant behavior is okay; it isn't. But it isn't indulgent to stop tearing yourself to shreds because you choose to evolve.

Reward yourself instead. If you catch yourself slumping in front of your computer, simply notice, say, "Aha," take a few deep breaths, and shift your position; enjoy the feeling of straightening your spine and bringing more oxygen into your lungs. If you catch yourself judging yourself in a Yoga class—*Everyone else is so fit; I'm a fat cow*—your reward might be simply to lift your shirt up and feel the air on your belly. That's a nice feeling. And it's a tiny, doable step—just feel the air. Continue to choose not to indulge in that judging behavior because that's what it is: indulging your internal sickness. Can you hang out with your belly for ten seconds without ripping yourself to shreds for not having six-pack abs?

Don't reward yourself in a way that will hurt you, like wolfing down chocolate cake or a bottle of wine. Instead, do something that gives you a momentary break. Take a walk to the water cooler and back. You don't have to do a Yoga pose, although that would be a great action. Instead of reaching for that cigarette, take deep breaths. Feel that there's something different that can arise when you break away from your own painful, habitual reactivity. What do you really feel under this surface feeling?

Avoid behavior that numbs you; you're looking for a reward that moves you into feeling. Honestly tell yourself, *That was really good! Congratulations! That was really skillful!* Offer yourself acknowledgment of the tremendous step you took by catching yourself in a bad pattern but *don't qualify it* with something like *Why didn't I do this ten years ago?* You weren't ready to do this ten years ago. Now is the time. Qualifiers damage us and deplete our energy.

You might also reward yourself with a five-minute massage on your foot, hand, belly, wherever. Step away from the computer and walk around the block and breathe some fresh air. Book a massage. Do something that has positive physical repercussions.

Catch your unconscious behavior over and over and over so you spend less time doing it. If you catch it one time out of ten, that's better than before. It takes time to repattern a whole neurological response. Rewarding yourself will speed up the process.

Take One Step Toward Healing

Even a tiny step can make an enormous difference in walking free from suffering. What's the one small step you can take to change an unhelpful pattern? If the answer is, "Nothing," you're not being creative enough.

Send your breath into the area that hurts and ask: *Who or what am I carrying here? What part of my life is stuck here?* Feel if your shoulders hurt. Shoulders have a lot to do with taking responsibility—often a responsibility that isn't yours to shoulder.

This is what I discovered with Wanda. Her shoulder would improve to a certain point, then plateau. We had to find out what else Wanda was carrying emotionally and psychologically. I asked her to take five or six deep breaths into her shoulder and ask: *What else am I carrying here?* It took a while, but we finally discovered that she was taking responsibility for her husband's back pain. (Women tend to put their needs second, so when they notice a tweaking or pain, they often ignore it and proceed with caring for others.) She was always trying to take care of him in a fussy, wifely way that made him really irritable, so he'd push her away verbally, which only added to the hurt. So now she had to catch another behavior; every time she felt the urge to caretake, she had to stop and breathe into her shoulders. Wanda had to change a whole dynamic with her husband. Her healing step was to back off and not irritate him with her fussy expressions of concern; it eased some of his grouchiness and got her out of her sacrificial, codependent pattern.

Do you feel stupid asking your body what it wants? We've been conditioned not to tap in to our body's wisdom, but we absolutely must. After a while, the body will respond. Sometimes we have to blast through years of deafness and numbness to our bodies before we'll hear back. Maybe we'll hear: *Don't push so hard* or *This relationship is making you sick* or *Ouch! What you're doing hurts!* If we've been responding with pain pills, it can take a while for that communication to get through.

Put your hand on the affected area, take a few breaths while you let your hand warm up, and ask for focus: *What do you need from me now? What step can I take to help?* Let the pain speak. You might get an odd little flash: *Rest. Stretch. Stop sitting with your legs crossed.* When I first started doing this, my self-talk would get in the way—*I can't do this; it's delusional talking to myself*—but when I'd shut up and listen, I'd usually hear something. Keep asking: *What do you need?* Get quiet and listen for a response. It might take a minute or two, or five or six days, but if you start to ask, you can regain that natural, healthy internal communication.

Get curious about what you can learn from your pain. A plant has a taproot—one primary, big, deep root—and lots of secondary roots. You don't have to find all those smaller roots, but you do need to find the taproot of your pain. Discover, go deep, and shift. What does the area in pain need? How can you give your pain a voice, and then offer it what it needs?

Automatic writing might help you figure things out. Sit down with your journal or keyboard and just let the thoughts flow. At first you might get boring stuff like *I need to pee* or *I need to do the dishes.* Keep going. Then read what you've written aloud to yourself. Put every ounce of feeling into your voice; let it resonate throughout your body. You might even experience physical symptoms while you're writing or reading aloud. Let's say I'm writing about someone I've loved and lost; I might feel a constriction in my heart, throat, and chest. As I read what I've written, I might put my hand on the constricted area and let the warmth of my hand comfort and encourage the emotion to come from that area. I can let my voice resonate from that area. What a difference from letting the storm rage!

HEALING EMOTIONAL PAIN

Holding on to anger, fear, or resentment can cause physical pain, but when we heal our emotional pain, our physical pain often subsides. Emotions need to be in motion in order for us to be healthy. We've got to move them and feel them and let them express themselves.

This is especially true with grief. In our culture, we don't know how to grieve properly; we get sick from the lack of it. Jerusalem has the Wailing Wall, a place to express grief. We need a place for allowing grief because it sits there in our cell tissue and depresses our immune system if we don't voice it. Grieving is looked down upon here. You can go ballistic at a funeral, but then you're supposed to be done. The ones who are stoic and shake everyone's hand are considered admirable even as they're imploding.

Take a courageous path: feel your grief and give it expression. Perhaps to someone close to you, it might seem like you're wallowing or drowning, but you do need to immerse yourself in your grief to move it out of your body. It's a sign of respect. Perhaps a parent has died, a friend has drifted away, or a child has left the nest. If you're grieving for a loved one you've lost, you're honoring that person by allowing those deep feelings of loss as well as anger and betrayal—*How could you leave me?*—to rise up and wash through you. Sometimes when we're grieving a person, we're also grieving the loss of a part of ourselves. Unexplored grief is like little glass shards that the body builds scar tissue around, and that can turn into sickness. Grief commonly shows up in the lungs as congestion, asthma, or other forms of entrapment. (In acupuncture, the area from the nipples to the collarbone is called the well of sorrow.) You can drown in your own grief when those areas aren't in motion.

Ceremonies—formal rituals, which might involve candles, tobacco, or sage—can be helpful for some people in expressing grief; for others it's just one more damn thing to do, an external that doesn't touch what's inside. For people who can imbue the ceremony with what's going on inside, it's very powerful. Ceremony may be beautiful, but in order to be healing, it has to move the stuck emotion. It's obvious when it happens: there's a lot of snot, a lot of strong feelings. You might have the shameful thought, *Oh, I'm just wallowing in poor pitiful me,* but if that's what it takes, go for it.

How long does it take to step out of grief? That's a very personal issue. When I was working on my own issues, friends really wished I would get over it because it made *them* uncomfortable. Some friends are able to tolerate your grieving more than others; that's why therapy can be a great thing, because that person is paid to sit through your pain and anger—"Here's a check. You walk me through this." Friends don't always have the tolerance and skill to navigate those deep waters. Everyone has their own "I've had enough" level. If friends have expressed theirs, don't take that as a judgment or allow self-mutilating thoughts like *I should be done grieving* or *I'm repulsive.* It's just that they need a break.

When my friend died, I struggled because I was with someone who was much closer to him, and I felt I wasn't entitled to grieve because she'd known him so much more. When I was able to articulate this to her, we both cried and got to share a Beauty moment, one that acknowledged both the pain and the release of pain that moved us both into healing. As we talked it out, a deer came up to us, very fearless. It was obviously what Native Americans call a Medicine moment—an important, pay-attention moment. You never know when you're opening a doorway to someone else's healing . . . or your own.

HEALING SPIRITUAL PAIN

Have you ever given up looking for something you yearned for—and you didn't even quite know what it was? Maybe the conscious part of you occupied with daily life didn't have time to keep searching, but some part of you was wordlessly crying out until you just had to deafen yourself to its cries because they were too painful and annoying. That was your own deep wisdom crying for connection to your Spirit.

Do you have insatiable yearnings? You're ravenous no matter how much you consume. No matter how many people you have sex with, you still feel lonely. No matter how much food you eat, you're never fully satisfied. Spiritual malaise or bereftness is a common condition, and the pain of being cut off from our Spirit often manifests itself as an indefinable yearning, which we typically try to fill with sex, alcohol, food, shopping, or other addictive behavior.

Do you know what it's like to feel your connection to your Spirit? When you have this kind of yearning, it's usually so deeply painful that you can't even discern it. You've walled it off because it's so unworkable. The yearning is with you so long that you seem to forget it as a way of coping. Sometimes this can be merciful numbing, but when it comes to tracking Spirit, we need to break down that silky membrane between our perceptions and the loss and emptiness. The first step in healing from the pain of addictive behavior is recognizing that the craving isn't for the alcohol or the person or whatever it is. Choose to take the Warrior's Step and hunt what that craving is really about—most likely your desperate need to connect to your Spirit.

PHYSICAL FOCUS:
EXERCISES FOR WALKING FREE OF PAIN

The Formula for Change will help you identify bad habits that cause or exacerbate physical pain. Now I want to share specific Yoga poses that will help with common problems. This will help you work to be free of pain *and* work pain-free. Learning how to be pain-free means paying attention to how you move and live in your body. For instance, continually checking in and straightening your spine and doing Shoulder Shrugs every hour while you're at your computer will help keep you pain-free. Or you can stay present and alert and conscious while doing a Yoga pose, paying attention to your personal edge—what you're capable of in that moment—instead of kinking your body because you think a pose needs to look a certain way.

Working pain-free means making intelligent choices. Let's say you're young and naïve and you make a New Year's resolution: *I want to get into better shape.* You've been a total couch potato, but from now on, you decide, you'll take a run every day. The first day you do five miles, and you're shredded; back to the couch for the rest of the year. Instead, walk a mile for a few days and gradually work up to running without pushing yourself into overexertion, which can lead to injury. Or perhaps you're recovering from abdominal surgery and you want to whip those abs back into shape, so you decide you'll do a few dozen rounds of Elbow to Knee (see page 58). Then you wake up screaming. Instead, start slowly, pulling your belly in with each exhale throughout the day. Then maybe work up to four repetitions of Elbow to Knee.

Pain is a signal. Sometimes it has to yell: *Pay attention, and change what you're doing!* It doesn't mean stop, necessarily, but it does mean deepen your breath, shift your weight, and give the area some physiological space so the pain can free up. Resting alone won't usually resolve the pain. When I work with professional athletes, they don't know how to use pain as a signal because they've been taught that to become extraordinary, they have to ignore or push through pain.

SIX STEPS TO FREEDOM FROM BACK PAIN

I want to pay special attention to back pain because 80 percent of Americans report experiencing it on a daily basis. Here I use a different approach from many other Yoga teachers. When you have damage in your back—say, a herniated disk—the muscles tend to splint, or harden, around it to immobilize the area. It's the body's intelligence trying to protect the lower back from further damage, but there's a more effective approach. You must replace the splinting with an equal action that creates strength and has more aliveness and intelligence. For example, do poses such as Elbow to Knee or moves like tucking the tailbone and telescoping the ribcage in order to give the area with the injury space and support. You need to understand what the body is doing so you can negotiate with it, protecting it without creating a locked-up quality.

Practice these six steps that will free you from back pain:

1 Identify the precise location of your back pain.

2 Breathe into that point of origin.

3 Create space in that point of origin.

4 Strengthen your core.

5 Use your legs to give you more support.

6 Learn to live spaciously internally.

Here are the steps in more detail.

Identify the Precise Location of Your Back Pain

This sounds obvious, but your body can fool you. Lower back pain could come from the collapse of your upper back. A lot of back pain comes from entrapment in the intestines. Here are some ways to read your back.

A lot of us have lower back pain because of constant compression of our spines. We don't sit or stand properly because we have poor posture and we don't use our abdominal muscles to support the lower back. If our abs are part of the no zone—an area we avoid because we think it's gross or fat—there's less and less support for the lower back. When you get your abdominals strong and responsive, then your back has more support.

To find out whether your back pain is coming from compression, do Back Traction pose. Lie on your back with your knees bent, feet flat on the floor under your knees. Then put your hands on top of your quads where your hips meet the front of the thighs. Push against your thighs, straightening your arms, and lift the chest away from the belly, tractioning the back out. Stay for five breaths. If this relieves your back pain, your problem is coming from compression. Doing Back Traction at least once a day will help. Making it a regular practice will help keep you pain-free.

Now lie belly down with a rolled-up towel or mat, six to ten inches in diameter, placed directly under your navel. If your back hurts in that position, the pain is coming from your intestines, colon, uterus, or other internal organs or from balled-up tension in that part of the body.

Frequently back pain can also be aggravated by intestinal blockage. How often do you have a bowel movement? You should poop as often as you eat meals. If you go once a day but eat three times a day, there's something wrong there. If you eat a poor diet, don't drink enough water, sit for half your lifetime, or have poor circulation, poop can clog up your intestines and narrow the channels; I call it shit shellac. This can show up as back pain. Changing your diet will clear it out eventually, and if you start doing abdominals, the shellac starts breaking up pretty quickly. Doing master cleanses or colonics can be somewhat helpful in the short term, but if you do them too often, your colon loses the ability to do peristalsis, and you get a whole new set of problems. Instead, eat a healthy diet with lots of whole grains and fiber-rich foods. Psyllium husk (Metamucil) can scour the shellac, and improving your breathing and posture will work wonders.

Sciatica pain typically runs through the buttocks muscles and/or down the back of the leg. If you think you have sciatica, try this test: stand up, tuck your tailbone down using your buttocks and abdominal muscles, and move your chest up. If that alleviates the pain and burning in your leg, you probably have sciatica. Doing forward bends with your legs straight to try to stretch them out is bad. Instead, lie on your back and bring your knees to your chest. Ab work will help, as will Bridge pose (see page 60) and Elbow to Knee (see page 58), which will contract and retrain the buttocks, the back of the thigh muscles, and the back. This will change how the sacrum sits in the body, which will take the pressure off the sciatic nerve and dissipate the pain. If you have sciatica, or hamstring or lower back pain, add this modification to Elbow to Knee pose: with your left knee bent and right leg straight, contract your right sit bone—the pointy bone at the bottom of your buttocks that you sit on—toward your tailbone. Do this healing variation each time you straighten the leg in Elbow to Knee.

Breathe into That Point of Origin

Once you've located your back pain's origin, close your eyes and take several deep breaths, focusing on bringing oxygen-carrying, cleansing breath to the damaged area, as I explained for Pigeon pose (see page 31). Breath is magic.

Create Space in That Point of Origin

Tuck your tailbone down to lengthen your spine. Then telescope your ribcage; pull your breath into the area so you can feel it expanding, making space. This can take pressure off the nerves and disks. If you put your hands on the sides of your ribs as you breathe, you can actually feel the expansion with every inhalation.

Strengthen Your Core

Make it a goal to teach the core to support the lower back. By core, I mean not just the abdominals (which are too often the sole focus), but also the chest and the upper, middle, and lower back as well as your buttocks muscles. The abdominal exercises, Elbow to Knee (see page 58), Lunges (see page 29), Bridge (see page 60), and Cross-Legged Side Bend (see page 61), are great for strengthening and toning your core. However, if you are pregnant, don't do abdominal exercises.

Use Your Legs to Give You More Support

Teach your legs to support the whole structure of your body for optimal function and spacious living. You'll find that by supporting your whole body with your legs, you also experience minimal wear on your joints. It is a stronger way to walk through life's challenges.

Bridge (see page 60) and standing poses such as Warrior I, Warrior II, and Extended Warrior Variation (see page 63) will strengthen your legs as they carry you on your life road.

Learn to Live Spaciously Internally

No matter how cramped your living quarters are, your spine and core can always be spacious. Learn to deep breathe and to sit and stand up without collapsing and compressing your back—a particular challenge for cubicle dwellers and keyboard jockeys. If you work on a computer a lot, your back and neck will get tight and you'll often have a lot of pain there. Neck Release pose, Shoulder Shrugs, and Spinal Twists (see pages 64–66) can free up the congestion and pain in that area, and they can be done while you're sitting in a chair.

YOGA POSES FOR A PAINFUL BACK

The following exercises, as well as Lunge (see page 29), work well for relieving pain in the back. Lunge is an amazing core declogger as well as a hip opener.

ELBOW TO KNEE

Elbow to Knee is a wonderful exercise for strengthening your core. Do it s-l-o-w-l-y and really pay attention to your breath. Start by lying on your back with your knees bent slightly less than ninety degrees, feet active and off the floor. Clasp your hands at the base of your skull, curling your forearms around your head. Press your lower back into the floor through all stages of this exercise. Inhale and lift your head and shoulders up. Hold your breath and lift your tailbone up. Then exhale, bringing both elbows toward your right knee. Straighten the left leg and pull your belly in. (This is a good place to add that healing variation of contracting the left sit bone toward the tailbone.) Inhale back to center, keep your head and shoulders up, hold your breath, and lift your tailbone. Exhale and reach both elbows toward your left knee. Straighten your right leg (contracting the right sit bone) and pull your belly in. Inhale back to center—keep head and shoulders up, hold breath, and lift tailbone. Repeat three to eight times.

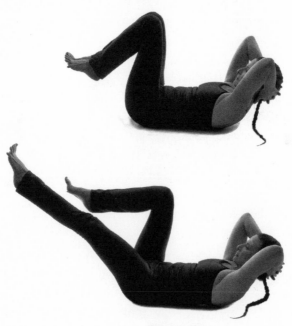

Elbow to Knee

ABS WITH A ROLL

You'll need a rolled-up mat or towel for this core strengthener. You get maximum benefits if you do it really slowly and pay attention to your breath and pulling your abs in. Lie on your back with the roll between your thighs against your crotch. Clasp your hands behind your head, forearms curled around your head, and lift your legs up straight. Inhale, press your lower back into the floor, hold your breath, lift your tailbone, and squeeze the mat between your thighs. Then exhale, curl your head and shoulders up, lift your tailbone a second time, squeeze the mat, and pull your belly in. Then inhale, rolling your shoulders, neck, and head back down to the floor. Repeat three to eight times.

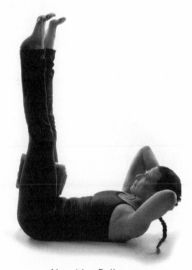

Abs with a Roll

FROG LIFTING THROUGH

This core strengthener works deeply. Lie on your back and clasp your hands behind your head, keeping the small of your back pressed to the ground. Lift your feet, bend your knees ninety degrees, and then separate your legs and turn your ankles out into a frog position, keeping your heels the same height as your knees. Inhale and curl your head and

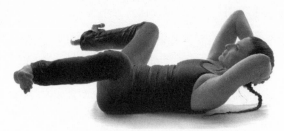

Frog Lifting Through

shoulders up. Exhale, curling your pubic bone toward your navel. Pull your belly in. Keep your head and shoulders up, inhale, and relax your pelvis down. Do five to eight rounds.

BRIDGE

I love Bridge because it strengthens the legs and starts to lighten up the gut while stretching out the back of the neck. The stretch on the back of the neck and the spread of the skull bones make my brain feel more spacious.

Lie on your back, knees bent and feet flat on the floor about a foot apart, with your heels aligned below your knees. Exhale and tilt your tailbone up. Then lift your pelvis and torso up, keeping your shoulders, neck, and head on the floor. Inhale and telescope your ribs toward your face. Exhale, press through your feet, and tilt your tailbone up even more. Take five to eight deep breaths. Keep your tailbone tucked as you come out of the pose.

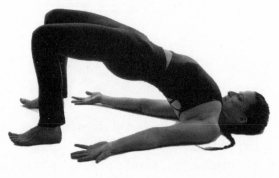

Bridge

CROSS-LEGGED SIDE BEND

Cross-Legged Side Bend stretches out the intercostal muscles, which improves the ability to take a deep breath. That changes every aspect of our life. And that's just the first part!

Sit on the floor with your legs comfortably crossed. Move your left hand straight out to the side, about a foot and a half from your left hip. Inhale, raise your right arm up over your right ear, with your palm facing the floor. Exhale and reach to the left. Relax your neck. Breathe and feel the stretch along your right side. Exhale, pulling your left shoulder down away from your left ear.

Second stage emphasizes release of the neck. To move into second stage, stretch your right arm to the right until your fingertips are twelve inches above the floor. Align your left ear over your left shoulder. Breathe deeply and slowly, relaxing your neck and jaw with each exhale. To release the pose, pull your right arm to the right to bring your torso upright. Now put your right hand down, leaving your head hanging. Use your left hand to cradle your head and lift it up. Stay in each stage for four breaths. Repeat on the other side.

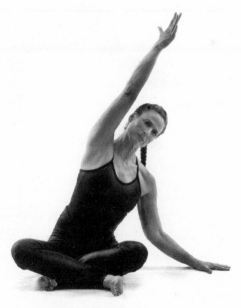

Cross-Legged Side Bend

WARRIOR I

Warriors are strong poses, and you can't wuss your way through them. Step four feet apart. Turn your right foot out and your left foot in about sixty degrees, keeping your heels aligned. Inhale and reach your arms up overhead, keeping your fingers active and stretching your ribs up. Exhale, bend your right front knee to ninety degrees, and tuck your tail-bone down. Square your hips toward your front knee. Take five deep breaths. Repeat on the other side.

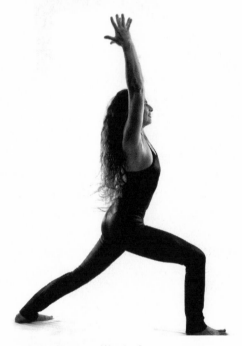

Warrior I

WARRIOR II

Step four feet apart. Turn your left foot out and your right foot slightly in. Then align the left heel with the arch on your right foot. Inhale, bring your arms straight out to the sides, feet and hands active, and tuck your tailbone down. Exhale and bend the front knee ninety degrees. Align your chin over your chest. Take five deep breaths. Repeat on the other side.

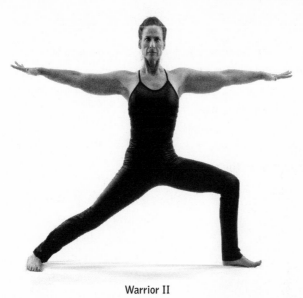

Warrior II

EXTENDED WARRIOR VARIATION

Come into Warrior II, place your left forearm onto your left thigh. Exhale, wrap your right arm behind lower back. Grab left thigh or the waistband of your pants. Pull the bottom shoulder away from the neck. Lift your ribs away from your left thigh by pushing through your left forearm. Relax your neck, feet active. Take five deep breaths. To release the pose, reach your right arm to the right side, pulling your torso up. Lift your head up last. Repeat on the other side.

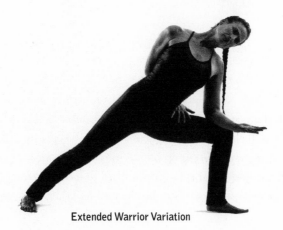

Extended Warrior Variation

YOGA POSES TO RELIEVE HURTING NECK AND SHOULDERS

NECK RELEASE POSE

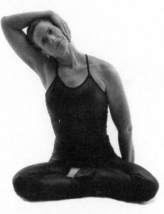

Neck Release Pose

Sit in a comfortable cross-legged position. Put your left hand under your left sit bone, palm down, with fingertips pointing toward the tailbone. Lean your head to the right and take a breath. Wrap your right arm up, over, and around your head so the fingertips are alongside the left jaw line. Keep the chest lifting up. (If this movement makes the pose too intense, just leave the left hand on the floor.) Lean your torso a bit to the right and take two breaths while relaxing the neck. Lower your head a couple inches, and breathe into the new area of tension in your neck for two more breaths. Lower your head another couple inches, breathe into the new stretch in your neck, and take two more breaths. Release your top arm down. Roll your chin toward your chest, and bring your torso back to center. Release the hand you're sitting on, leave the head hanging, and take a breath into the back of the neck. Place your hand on your forehead, inhale, and lift the head up. Repeat on the other side.

SHOULDER SHRUGS IN WARRIOR II

Step four feet apart. Turn your right foot out and your left foot slightly in. Then align the right heel with the arch on your left foot. Bring your arms straight out to the sides, fingers active, exhale and bend the right front knee ninety degrees, and tuck your tailbone down. Align your chin over your chest. Now you're in Warrior II pose. Keep your arms hanging and relaxed. Inhale, ballooning breath into your upper back. Hold your breath as you shrug your shoulders up and pull them straight back. Exhale, squeezing your upper shoulder blades together. Drag them down.

Then release. Inhale, broaden your upper back. Exhale, squeezing your mid-shoulder blades together and dragging them down. Relax and inhale into your upper back. Exhale, squeezing the bottom tips of your shoulder blades together, dragging them down. Release, then inhale. Repeat two more times.

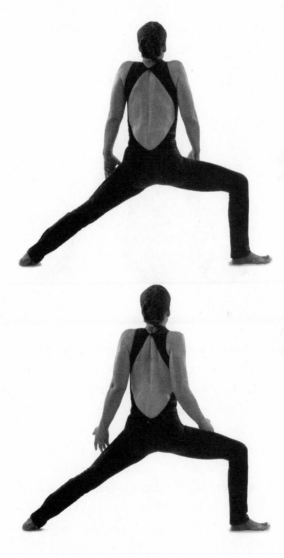

Shoulder Shrugs

SPINAL TWIST

Sit cross-legged. Put your left hand on your right knee and your right hand behind your sacrum, fingertips on the floor pointing away from the sacrum. Inhale and telescope your ribs up. Keeping the lift, exhale and twist to the left, aligning your chin over your chest. As your flexibility allows, increase the twist with each exhale. Hold for five breaths. Cross your legs the other way and do the other side.

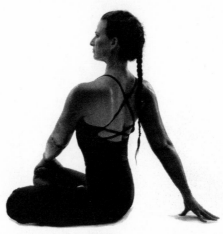

Spinal Twist

Pain, whether physical, emotional, or spiritual, need not be a constant in your life. You can always choose to develop a different relationship to it, so if you cannot walk free of it completely, you can liberate yourself from the suffering you've attached to it. That is a walk of freedom.

3

TRUTH SPEAKING:
BUILDING THE WARRIOR'S HEART

MAYA TOOK a meditative puff on her cigarette and then lit one for me. We stood together in the backyard, this housekeeper and I, smoking and talking. "You know what your mother is?" she asked me. "She's the wild sow that ate its own young. What the hell is wrong with these people that they can't see what a monster she is? And your father? He's an asshole."

I could barely breathe; I was so shocked and thrilled. At six, I was already sick of people always telling me about my wonderful mother, what a hardworking school teacher she was. Once she even won a Golden Apple Award for her efforts. Whenever I was chewed out in the principal's office for mouthing off again, I'd be warned about "the repercussions of my actions on my mother's reputation." She was teaching kids my age, and I could picture her being so sweet to them, but when she got home, it was like she'd given everything she had at the office, and all she had left for me was threats and hitting. I was sick of hearing my father praised for his efforts as a social worker, helping kids get placed in foster care, so committed to improving the lot of others. Behind closed doors, he never stepped in when Mother went off on bitter rants or came after me. Life at home was a secret hell—or so I thought. Maya was a silent but power-ful witness to it all.

A slender African American woman with close-cropped hair, Maya wasn't big on demonstrations of affection, although every now and then she'd sling her arm around my shoulder. More often she'd simply stand with me in the kitchen, stony-faced and impassive, while my parents had one of their screaming fights in the next room. She couldn't step in and defend me when my mother attacked me, but she'd tell me what she thought afterward, calling my mother a mad dog and a bitch.

I'm sure some people think it wasn't a great idea to give a cigarette to a six-year-old, but I lived for the smoke breaks with Maya. They were the only honest discussions I ever had as a child, and Maya was the only adult who made me feel safe. Observing the filth that constantly piled up between her cleaning visits, my parents' increasingly virulent fights, and the general level of insanity in my home, Maya would wrinkle up her round face and whisper, "You're not crazy; *they're* crazy." Maybe I wasn't an evil demon seed, as my mom said, after all. Maya would give me ad-vice on how to handle life at home, but more importantly, she just lis-tened to me. I still remember that nicotine rush, which I associate with the letting down of shields. What sweet relief, after all those lies, lies, lies, to hear Maya speak the truth. Years later, when I first connected to Native American Medicine and learned how to use tobacco to pray, to speak heart-to-heart with another, I had to laugh; Maya with her ciga-rettes had been my first Medicine teacher.

Maya was my first Truth Speaker, someone who spoke from her heart and told the truth with great compassion. I wondered if I could use what I'd learned from Maya with the kids down at the stables. I wasn't ex-actly craving friendship, just some kind of interaction. The other stable brats—social rejects like me—were all in their teens and twenties, run-ning wild, beating each other up, picking locks and hot-wiring cars, gal-loping the rent horses out on the nearby golf course and tearing the turf into shreds. Six years younger than the next youngest one, I was reli-able entertainment for them. The older kids stole alcohol and drugs, and they found it amusing to give them to me. I was a mascot, a disposable toy to them—something to dump into the sharp-edged horse trough or toss off a haystack. But they were all I had. I tried to assure myself a position in the pack by becoming even more wild and unpredictable than they were, a kind of insane jester who threw down the biggest dares, who never balked at any challenge.

For some reason, though, these much older kids sensed something beyond my tough kid act. They started coming to me with their problems, most of which were out of my league. I was ten or eleven. What did I know about who was sleeping with whom, or why? If they told me something that I couldn't relate to in terms of life experience, I'd start listening differently. It was as if their words dropped down inside a well. There'd be a silent, pregnant moment, and then a response would come from someplace deep within me. I wouldn't think about it; I'd just say it. It was weird—and I liked it. Giving advice was better than being thrown around. Soon even the ones who'd roughed me up the most were coming to me for my words of wisdom.

Renee, for instance, was having boyfriend trouble. She was an oddity for the stable: a girly girl who wore tons of eyeliner, her hair ratted up and her clothes hugging her body in the style of the day. She was complaining to me about how much she and her boyfriend, Ray, were fighting. What should she do? The answer came up from the well: "Ask him what he needs." How strange was that? This was the late sixties. No one was asking teenagers about their needs; certainly no one had asked Ray. But it did the trick. Soon Ray was coming to me for advice too.

At the same time, my defensive shields were impregnable. They were so much a part of me that I thought they *were* me. In my mouth, truth was a really sharp weapon, something I'd use to outmaneuver anyone who got aggressive with me or seemed superior. Like Harry, who was just a little bit softer than the rest of us brats, a little more "moneyed." Maybe somebody even loved him. I put him in my sights. When I found out he was scared of Poncho, this dun-colored horse that was constantly spooking at the ghosts in his mind, I'd throw Harry's fearfulness and lack of experience in front of the whole group, like feeding a wounded fish to a shark tank: "You're afraid of Poncho? You're eight years older than me, and I can ride him. He can dump you anytime." Fearfulness around horses was the kiss of death in the stables. The gang loved my razor tongue—until it was them getting cut. If someone crossed me, I'd take the secret they'd shared with me and fling it at their feet in front of everybody. I used the truth irresponsibly, shooting it like an arrow with intent to wound, yet also to pierce the emotional infections we all had— even then I was attempting to heal. I couldn't trust anyone, and they couldn't trust me.

Other than Maya and Nick, the only ones who told me the truth were the horses. When a horse is pissed at you, it'll try to kick or bite the hell out of you. When a horse likes you, you can feel the affection radiate from it. Horses were the only living things I loved without reserve—and they, in turn, accepted me. I'd spend hours in their quiet company. The pecking order of the horses in the corral made sense. Some horses buddied up, standing head to tail and rubbing their teeth on each other's backs, swishing the flies off each other. This equine social system was the first model of relationship for me. With the gang, I was always wired up or drunk or high or fighting for my life with my fists or words. The horses seemed to have it all figured out so easily. And if one stepped out of line, a quick bite restored order. Horses fascinated me.

Nick let each of us brats pick a favorite rent horse as a special pet, someone to give extra attention to, and if there wasn't too much work to do, maybe take for a ride. I picked Span, the ugliest horse in the stable. She was an old swayback with lumps on her legs, a funny knobby Roman-nosed head, and a completely unredeeming gait. She was a safe choice because no one else wanted her. I'd already learned that whenever I wanted something, it would be taken away from me. But no one would take Span; she was a throwaway, like me.

Span taught me even more about relationships. I figured maybe she would like me if I liked her. At first, when I started brushing Span and giving her carrots and putting medicine on her legs, she was a pretty dejected thing—two steps from dog food. (The other kids called her Spam.) She had that dead look in her eyes; hanging out with her was like playing with a smelly statue with sores on it. Then little by little, her eyes started to come alive. One day I was brushing her when she turned to me and lightly touched her nose to me as if to say, *Hey, I noticed you were there.* I didn't have the words for it then, but I could sense I was bringing her Spirit back. Maybe that could happen for me too. I was afraid to care for Span because I was sure she'd be taken from me, but I began to anyway.

I have a feeling that this was Nick's plan from the beginning. He was one of the first humans to notice me with any interest or affection. I'd be scrapping with the older kids, and I'd turn and see him watching silently. He saw that I needed to learn to care, so he left that ugly old mare for me. Both kid and horse began to heal. When there's that affectionate bond, something else develops in the four-foot—this is what Native Americans call four-footed animals—*and* the two-foot person. All of us brats had raw wounds. Caring for our special pets was balm for the heart. It soothed our wounds. It also grew something inside of us, gave us a place for affection and touch—things that should have been a part of everyone's experience but had never been part of ours. Maybe that's why I'd hated Harry. Somebody *had* petted him. Somebody *had* cared about him. Caring for Span allowed something to grow inside me that had never had a proper environment before.

Azusa Canyon Stables was such a refuge for me over those years, sometimes literally the only roof over my head, the place where I learned to train and care for horses, the laboratory for my study of relationships. Then a series of small disasters hit us—bad fires and heavy rains gradually sent most of our customers to other stables. The place was dying by inches. Then one day a huge flood swept over the whole canyon, including the stables, burying it in mud from the nearby barren, scorched mountains.

In a flash, the place where I'd started to bring myself to life was totally destroyed. All the roads had been washed out, the stables drowning in mud. I stood on a slurry of muddy rock, watching helicopters drop bales of hay down to the horses trapped on the other side of the raging, swollen river. I felt whatever little glimmer of aliveness that had been growing in me get duller and duller. Old Harry, an elderly guy living nearby, had suffocated in the mud; I heard he'd refused to evacuate when they were trying to rescue people. Maybe he'd decided there was nothing to live for. I don't know if Span made it out. The only thing that kept me from giving up completely like Old Harry was that I had a pinto horse called Caprice trapped inside those stables. She was the first horse I ever really owned. If I could just get on her back, I told myself, I'd be all right. I came up with the crazy idea of rescuing my horse.

I forded the river and emerged battered and bruised to fight my way into the tack room. Everything there was ruined by mud and water, useless. I grabbed up an old cracked bridle and rode Caprice bareback. I urged her into the currents. It was terrifying, but I felt like I was fighting for both of our lives. I somehow got Caprice safely to the other side but then realized I had no idea where to go from there.

Certainly not back to school. By tenth or eleventh grade, I'd already dropped out. I remember one day the teacher asked me to stay after class. *Now what?* I thought, *What am I going to get chewed out for this time?* He handed me an evaluation form so I could assess what I thought of the gifted classes I was in. *Gifted classes?* I'd had no idea; no one had ever mentioned it. I sat there, filling out this ridiculous true-false questionnaire when I looked out the window at a tree. As I watched, a leaf broke off of the tree and fluttered to the ground. When it landed, a strong epiphany hit me: *I'm wasting my life. From branch to ground is how much time I have left.* I got up out of my chair and walked out of the building; I never went back to high school. I fought the whole school district and won the right to enter an experimental adult school that let me fulfill my high school requirements. That was huge. This was a different kind of fight; I wasn't fighting against being thrown into a trough, and I wasn't yelling back at a stupid teacher; I was standing up for something meaningful for me, and the fact that I won changed something inside me.

After Caprice I bought a half-breed Arabian foal, one of the oldest and greatest horse lineages in the world. He was too young to ride, so I taught him how to carry a saddle, respond to a bit, follow voice signals, and pull a cart, so he was half-trained. I finally got myself a chance to work in a show barn under a guy named Mike Nielson, an internationally respected trainer of hunters and jumpers. I sold my half-Arab to buy a horse I'd found neglected in an outside stall. She was a blue-eyed cream horse with pink skin covered with scabs; hence her nickname, Scabby. She looked like a unicorn that had dropped her horn. I named her Chelsey Morning after the Joni Mitchell song "Chelsea Morning."

She'd let me sleep with her in her stall; I'd snuggle right up against her foreleg and neck.

I was told there was no room in the show world for a pink horse, my magical hornless unicorn; still, I was showing her a lot and I was winning. Mike told me I'd only go so far with her. "She's a good girl, but the wrong color." I hated selling Chelsey, but I needed a conventional-colored horse if I was going to win at larger national competitions. So I bought copper-colored Squirrel and gave him the show name Where Does It Hurt? (In the horse world, horses commonly have a nickname and a longer, grander show name. Squirrel's show name came from a movie whose title seemed particularly apt to me.) He was a young thoroughbred who was completely wild, agile, and beautiful. I got him cheap because no one else could ride him. It was my dream to be a horse trainer like Mike. My plan was to train Squirrel and thereby prove my abilities to Mike and work my way up to being his acknowledged assistant.

In the meantime, though, my official title at the horse shows was groom. I'd sleep in the tack room and wake up at three A.M. to start cleaning and feeding the horses and mucking the stalls. I'd get the horses ready for show and ride them as needed. But if I got invited to a celebratory dinner after someone won a ribbon, I'd risk embarrassing Mike—I was too weird and hostile; I didn't know how to eat at a table with silverware. Once, after I was trying to saw through a steak and it flipped into the lap of a woman dubbed Best Dressed in Covina, Mike joked, "God, I can't take you anywhere." I knew it'd take me a long time to make it as his assistant.

I somehow wrangled myself a job at a ranch that bred Morgans, a particularly kid-friendly breed, out in Hesperia, in the desert. I was being hired as a trainer for the first time. The ranch owner offered me terms that were so hideous, even I knew it: twenty-five dollars a week plus a place where I could live with my horse and a dog that had somehow attached himself to me. I took the job; once I turned eighteen, I'd be out of the junior category, so I needed to prove myself as a recognized horse trainer as soon as possible. Without bothering to mention it to my parents, I loaded up my beat-up old Vista Cruiser and hightailed it out to the desert with Squirrel in tow.

Cleaning and feeding and training the horses in the desert was exhausting, backbreaking work. You want to talk about an education? Try pulling foals out of their mothers in the middle of the night all by yourself. I was also helping with the breeding. Watching two horses mate was like being in the middle of a storm. The owner and her girlfriend would come to the ranch once a month to check in, and there was a rent-a-kid from some horrible youth prison camp nearby who'd come around very rarely. But basically I was on my own. The pay was so crappy that I couldn't afford to eat every day. Somehow—and I don't even remember how—I managed to scrounge up cigarettes and alcohol. Sometimes I'd eat some of the horse food just to fill my belly. I felt guilty taking the horses' feed, but I was starving.

Once a month I'd go into town to pick up supplies. After my shopping, I'd go to a diner and order the same thing—a ham and cheese omelet, my big feast for the month. Every time I went back, the portion would get bigger and bigger and bigger. Sometimes the waitress would pass by my table and just slide a couple extra pieces of toast onto my plate. I'd look at her, try to smile, not able to express the thanks I felt in my heart. That unsolicited generosity marked me. Like Nick and Span, those people at the diner planted a seed for something different, something of beauty to grow inside me.

I'd exchange a couple words with the rent-a-worker, but I just didn't want to deal with speaking. Out in the desert, I pretty much stopped talking, and then I stopped thinking in words. Snakes, vultures, horses, coyotes, and my dog were my companions. I'd sit out at night beneath the vast velvet blackness of space and stars and howl out the anguish of my heart with the coyotes. That was some really damn clear Truth Speaking. The coyotes were always up for a good sing-along. With the horses, I would nicker, snort, and make other horse sounds as best I could. When I spoke in their language, it removed me from the human world—which felt distorted, lying, and insane, where I was starving and unloved and forever struggling without succeeding. Communicating with the critters gave me a level of solace that I never got anywhere else.

Ironically, going into silence was how I, this numbed-out alcoholic kid, learned to Speak Truth. I wasn't talking to anybody, but I was communicating truthfully—with the animals. I know it may sound crazy, but there's just no lying. In the horse and coyote worlds, there's a vast vocabulary without words; they do so much communicating with their bodies that sounds are almost like exclamation points. I learned to communicate with them, as well as with hawks and snakes, by sending out pictures from my mind and some kind of energy from inside my torso.

In the desert during the hottest part of the day, doing heavy physical labor outdoors can be deadly. Sunstroke and dehydration are the main culprits. I'd go to the shadows of a little hill during those times and lie on flat rocks that warmed me without baking me. I soon discovered that rattlesnakes liked them too. There was something really comforting about hanging out with them; they had a kind of relaxed hypervigilance. I studied their signals, how they flicked their tongues and moved their heads around when they were sensing their world. They conversed through movement and contact and rattles. They wouldn't seek out conversations with me; I didn't speak the same language. I'd send a silent message out to them—*Hey, I'm here! Don't bite me.* They usually didn't respond. Once in a great while, though, I'd get a snake to answer me. I'd get a feeling in my head and body that I was accepted. Hanging out with the snakes taught me to become still, because being restless by a rattler could be deadly.

Those snakes fascinated me. I could see that they weren't just pretty, they were astonishingly *beautiful*—they had a lot of sparkle. I was doing what the Native Americans call seeing in Beauty. Beauty is fires and floods and scorching sun and the patterns on a rattlesnake's skin. To feel real Beauty on this earth—the struggles as well as the lovely surfaces and depths—is the most amazing thing.

I was such a deeply damaged thing back then. Communing with the horses, howling with the coyotes, and being in the silent, accepting presence of the snakes was how I began to thaw my frozen heart. I wasn't yet able to show my pain to anyone else—*I'm hurt* was a secret. Loneliness wasn't a problem—the times when my mother neglected me were sadly the best part of our relationship. Being alone, away from humans, was a relief. Still, in no way could I show how hurt I'd been. In the animal world, when you show pain, you're basically saying, *Hey, I'm your lunch. Come get me.* Humans have the same instinct to prey on what's vulnerable.

I could at times begin to feel a whole toxic storm inside me, but I didn't yet know exactly what had happened to me. I remembered my mother's physical violence, her switching, but it didn't seem to justify the vastness of the storm inside me. I would figure that out later. There was something that had happened that was so terrible that I couldn't remember it. I began to perceive that there was a big steel-plated door that was every kind of shut—dead-bolted, chained—and behind it was something that would obliterate me if it ever got out.

Feeling that visceral truth was the beginning of becoming a Truth Speaker.

SPEAKING WHAT MATTERS

Truth Speaking—speaking from a place of deep honesty and compassion—propels us into a very rich field of feeling. Every time we speak the truth, it shudders through the cobwebs and dimness in our lives, tapping back in to the Beauty in our world, in ourselves, and in each other. How incredibly sweet it is to be able to talk about what's really important, stepping out from behind our facades and the little stupid conversations that we're taught are a necessary social lubricant. When we Speak Truth to each other, once we get past the shock, it kindles the desire to hear the truth coming back at us.

I encourage you to take this wild and exciting path of Truth Speaking because it's unfathomably rich. It's also risky. But what are you risking? All the facades that make your life dull and boring and complacent. By speaking the truth, we learn the difference between our authentic self and our facade. If we put our little masked self out there, the horror is that other people might accept and end up making love to it, while we starve and die of neglect behind it. It's much richer to interact genuinely with the world.

When you speak the truth, it feeds and brightens your Spirit. When you don't, it dims your Spirit. Don't you want to live in a way that brightens your Spirit? To take a deep breath and feel what's rocketing and roiling around in your core? What a delight!

STEPPING ONTO THE BRAVE-HEARTED PATH
WITH A WARRIOR'S HEART

The first step to Truth Speaking is opening our hearts. Sometimes we resist this because we think it means that anything and anyone can come in and do us harm. There's a difference between an open heart, which can feel, process, and stay steady, versus a stuck-open-window heart, which lets all sorts of crap fly in.

I encourage you to develop a Warrior's Heart—an open heart that is responsive and reflexive, meaning that when something comes in and touches it, the heart responds and bounces right back. Most people's hearts, however, are flabby—atrophied and weak. Something comes in—love, hate—and the flabby heart energetically folds around it and encapsulates it. When we curl around the pain, that's when it embeds. A heart has to be healthy to feel, respond, and flex. Empaths—people who feel other people's feelings—especially need to be able to feel the world without letting its woes root deep within them.

A really big part of the Brave-Hearted Path is being able to respond from a Warrior's Heart while using the discernment of the heart, brain, gut, and every other power and intelligence center of the body. We're mostly taught to respond from our intellect, which is a very small part of our faculties, so we end up making decisions that aren't fully informed, which are usually mistakes. It's like taking action after collecting the votes of only two people on a council of eight; you're only using part of your resources, which isn't wise.

Truth Speaking means speaking from the heart with honesty and compassion. When I say from the heart, I don't mean to gush—as in, "I love you, man!" I believe the heart has a number of attitudes; it has its own wisdom and compassion, and it will guide you in Truth Speaking. *Compassion* is a funny word; we think of it as being kind to someone else. I don't agree. As I see it, compassion needs to encompass ourselves, the person we're dealing with, *and* the situation. It means looking at and feeling for a resolution that feels most correct by the standards of the heart, mind, and gut. In learning a truth about myself, I found that I could be completely honest but without compassion for the other person and the situation. Words were used as weapons and shields. I needed to develop some generosity of heart to cultivate compassion.

Truth Speaking also means fighting for what's right. I'm not talking about fighting with hands or guns; I'm talking about taking a stance in your truth as best you know it and speaking from that place of integrity.

When you act with a Warrior's Heart, you understand that it's not about being right versus being wrong. Being right isn't necessarily a win. Nor is simply giving in to the other person—*Okay, fine, you're right. Let's do it your way.* That breeds resentment and imbalance. As a friend described it, acting with a Warrior's Heart means "having to think with your heart and feel with your brain."

SPIRITUAL FOCUS:
EXERCISES TO TONE A FLABBY HEART

BEGINNING TO THAW: FEELING TRUTH

Building heart strength can free us from past pains and grievances—and help us keep our hearts open no matter what comes our way. Speaking Truth with a Warrior's Heart—whether to a friend, a coworker, a romantic partner, or ourselves—can thaw the heart we've closed down because of great pain.

When I was young, I stopped crying at a very early age. I'd be beaten if I cried. Learning to disconnect from my feelings kept my sanity intact. It was both the way I was conditioned as well as a very powerful defense mechanism. My earliest lesson about love was: don't ever say what you care about because it'll be used against you. To drive that one home, someone once killed a kitten in front of me and said, "If you love something, it dies horribly." One of my greatest healing miracles is triumphing over that vicious conditioning and learning to love.

I spent most of my early life looking to get numb and stay numb. I liked the numbness of alcohol and the burn when I smoked cigarettes or got high. I liked to stand out in the freezing cold or the searing desert heat. It was all about becoming impervious—to the elements, to being kicked by a horse, to any kind of pain. But I also became impervious to my own feelings. My intellect would be there, present and accounted for, listening, responding, but my emotions were unavailable to other people. I could barely access them myself—the ultimate disconnect. How often did I hear from my Yoga teachers, "You must first love yourself before you can love others"? That's a myth. If I had to do that, I'd be dead. What can someone in that position feel? Learning love came in steps for me.

If you've numbed yourself against pain for a long time, you need to bring yourself back to life gradually, with great care. If you're emotionally atrophied—perhaps because you're in a loveless relationship or stuck in a mindless desk job—you've got to start small, very small. You have to build up a reservoir of self-respect and care before you can give to someone else or you'll be giving from a place of emptiness, which is one of the accepted disorders of our society.

I want you to practice feeling. For example, close your eyes, put your hands over your heart, and take several deep, full-body breaths into your heart. Feel your heart respond to your breath. That's a really good step.

Can you rub your foot and allow yourself to feel the pleasure of it? Your assignment: every night before you go to sleep, look at your clock, and for one minute rub your foot and luxuriate in how good that feels. You don't have to be a reflexologist or a professional massage therapist; just rub your foot and stay with the feeling the whole time. Then you can buy a beautiful-smelling massage oil and rub your hands and feet. Practice enjoying the basic language of touch.

The contact with the horses and the other animals out in the desert kept my heart alive. For you, the process of thawing may likewise begin not with another human, but with a plant or an animal, which can be easier to connect to.

Go sit with a tree. Touch it. Feel its bark; look at its patterns really closely. Maybe you can feel its life force slowly pulsing through it. No matter how damaged you are, you can put your fingers or your cheek on that tree and take that first step.

If you can't get to a tree, can you commune with your houseplant? Can you practice feelings with your pet? When you reach out to that other living being, whether plant or animal, you're unshielding your heart, allowing it space to expand and strengthen.

Is it a mistake to open your heart before you strengthen it? No. In order to teach your heart resilience, you have to let it out of its box so your heart learns to breathe, flex, get on with it.

SPEAKING TRUTH TO YOURSELF

When you feel sufficiently thawed, take the next step in Truth Speaking—look inside yourself and feel, think, and perceive what injury or issue needs to be addressed, what it is that you really need to hear or want to say. This requires a team effort between mental and emotional processes.

It's not always easy to discern what truth wants to emerge. Our truths grow as we grow. If you're looking at just the trunk of an elephant, your truth might be that you see a wrinkly snake. As you see more of the critter, your perception will grow because you have more information, but your first perception wasn't wrong; it was the best you could do at the time. Honor that. Give yourself permission to make mistakes and learn from them, a necessary part of the process.

When a truth comes to you through intuition, it usually comes out in a flash as a whole concept. When you're trying to get to the truth of a situation by thinking your way there bit by bit, it might come in pieces. Whenever I've had epiphanies (whole revelations), they've come through intuition, although I've sometimes been able to jump-start the process by thinking. You will learn to keep checking in with your body's wisdom, using breath and feeling, to know when you're getting to the truth; that's the Brave-Hearted Path.

So sit, get quiet, take at least three deep breaths, and ask yourself: *What's going on with me?* Perhaps you can sense an uncomfortable feeling that's ready to come out. Or maybe you've come to a decision about a situation that's not working for you anymore. When you've arrived at the truth, you'll feel a resonance throughout your whole body. It's like a little energetic orgasm. I literally feel my blood quicken, which has a direct, enlivening effect on my heart.

Sit with this truth, then ask yourself: *What's the most healing action I can take as a next step?* Please notice that I used the word *healing*, not *loving* or *kind*. That's because many of us—especially women—have been silently conditioned to become what I bluntly refer to as Sacrificial Whores; we'll do or say something that makes us feel we've been nice or kind, so that people will still love us. That's not wise, and it may not be the most compassionate action in the situation. Some truths are hard, yet they must be acknowledged. So after you've asked for that next healing action, take a deep breath, relax, and listen to what comes up. If you get silence, maybe that's exactly what you need to give yourself time for. Can you honor what comes up and then do it, even if only for a few moments?

Recently I was having trouble with my thyroid gland, which sits just beneath the throat; it plays a huge role in regulating metabolism and energy levels. In Yoga tradition, the fifth or throat chakra is the seat of self-expression. When we Speak Truth, it comes in part through the throat. So when I developed hypothyroidism and lumps on my thyroid, it was easy to see how that tied into some issues I was working on. For one thing, I've found that it's very hard for me to admit that something's wrong with me, that I'm in need of healing. After all, I've been teaching Yoga for more than thirty-five years; aren't I supposed to be the healer, not the patient? But hell, ever since I've been alive, there's been something wrong with me that I've had to learn to deal with: being crippled, epilepsy, drug addiction, alcoholism, bulimia, smoking, you name it. My thyroid imbalance prompted me to do some Truth Speaking to myself. I asked that part of my body what it needed. The answers were that I needed to speak more about what compels me and what is most precious to me. And I needed to learn how to rest on a regular basis. As of today, I'm still working on these two truths. I understand now that as I continue to heal myself, I become a better healer.

TRUTH SPEAKING WITH OTHERS

Speaking the truth often feels very scary, especially if you're sharing something that might put another person on the defensive, such as, "You hurt me when you do this." When I feel the need to Speak Truth, the first thing I do is start breathing deeply through my core. Next I get my feet active, tuck my tailbone, activate the muscles in my thighs and pelvis, and get as steady as I can. I know that a storm is brewing inside me because I'm about to shred one of those veils that have kept me hidden. I'll go over what I want to say, picturing and feeling what it would be like to speak it, which also helps me get steady. Sometimes I can focus and breathe and get the words right out; other times I stumble over my words and feel like a fool. Sometimes I'll ask for feedback from whomever I'm speaking to so I'll know I got my message across.

When you first start to Speak Truth, it may come pouring out, like verbal puke. Be gentle with yourself; you'll make slow, steady progress, moving from a single sentence to Speaking Truth for a full day.

As with any new skill, you need to practice. Pick a friend you have some affection for. Have a Truth Speaking conversation with him or her. Deliberately take your shields down. Touch a safe place on the other person—the shoulder or arm—and let yourself actually feel what you feel for your friend for a little unshielded moment. Find out if you're ready for a bigger step—maybe you'll have an unshielded conversation.

Walk with me through this example from my own life. My first husband, John, had said something nonchalant and careless about sex; I can't even remember what it was. At the time, I was in the therapeutic process of unraveling my childhood sexual abuse. Everything felt personal and wounding, especially around sex. I went into full-blown trigger mode about his comment, howling inside, *How could you? Don't you know?,* as though he were supposed to be able to walk through my internal minefield even though *I* didn't even know how to do that. I wanted to run, I wanted to attack him, and I wanted to die—all within about thirty seconds. I shut down so violently that I felt like I was being strangled. I couldn't say a word.

It took me three weeks to sort out my issues. Part of it was about control—I'd been so hurt and out of my own control as a child, so brainwashed, that I'd lost my power of speech. I'd have crazy rules in my head like *John, every night you're supposed to stay up all night and watch over my dreams and make sure* they *don't get me* (and that was one of the more minor rules). This was hard to admit to myself. I spent those three weeks in turmoil. I'd wake up and find cuts in my palms from my fingernails digging into them. My back was spasming, my neck was kinking, my headaches were blazing, and my legs were crumbling.

After three weeks, I finally choked out my first communication. I sought John out and told him, "When you said that thing about sex, it really hurt me." The truth was that I'd just ripped off all this emotional scar tissue with therapy and I was a big, bloody, oozing mess, and I was so sensitive that even just the wind of his passage hurt.

John's first response was, "I have no idea what you're talking about." I had a huge internal reaction to that: *Oh, my needs don't matter.* That wasn't the truth of it, but that was what was triggered in me. I wanted to walk out, but I made myself stay and explain.

"Why didn't you tell me at the time?" John asked, a sensible question.

I went from ashamed to angry and defensive. I just blurted out, "I'm telling you *now*."

After what felt like a year of discussion, John finally admitted, "You're right. That *was* a careless comment. I wasn't thinking, but I didn't mean it as a dig."

That was all I got. I wanted a bigger response from him, one that matched my huge reaction. But John was speaking his own truth; this hadn't been a big deal for him, even though for me it was a huge battle that took everything I had to fight. This was a powerful lesson for me: to allow the listener the freedom to react or respond in whatever way he or she will.

I realized later that this Truth Speaking had a lot of small but significant wins: I hadn't obeyed the shutdown. I hadn't walked away. I hadn't shot my little arrows of truth into John's sensitive parts as a diversionary tactic. I persisted in seeing the conversation through instead of telling myself, *Oh, never mind. It doesn't matter.* Before that, I could fight for anyone else's cause to the death, but not my own, so it was a win to fight for myself. And it was a win to realize that John's reaction wasn't my responsibility to control. *My* reaction was my responsibility. It was a relief to take my psychic control off of John—so exhausting—and let him do whatever he was doing. (I have to relearn this lesson a lot.)

TALKING CIRCLE

A talking circle is a great way to practice Truth Speaking. Traditionally, that's a ceremony in which people sit in a circle and pass around a ceremonial object—a stick, most commonly—and people have the power to speak what's uppermost in their heart when they're holding the stick. While the stick holder talks, absolutely no interruptions are permitted until the stick holder is completely finished speaking his truth. Then that person says, "Aho," or "Amen," or another word that signifies that he is finished. Then he passes the stick to the next person in the circle. This continues until everyone has talked out whatever issue is under discussion. The group may or may not solve a problem; this is about giving everyone a voice. (I jokingly call it a listening circle, since you spend much more time listening than talking.)

When I do a talking circle in my teacher training, I limit everyone to three minutes and we only go around the circle once because I want my students to learn to Speak Truth from the heart in a succinct way. If you want to do a talking circle, the rules to honor are: don't interrupt anyone, speak the truth as best you can from your heart, listen whole-heartedly, and stay in the circle until it's done. It helps to have a topic initially to guide the focus, which may change as people speak. If something is burning in your heart, this is the arena to speak it. This may seem like a long, time-consuming process, but it's actually a shortening of the way because each person can empty out her thoughts and feelings, when in an ordinary meeting situation these might get backlogged for weeks or years.

It's amazing to learn to do a talking circle. You can set it up as a group or do it one on one. Gather your group. State the rules, declare the topic, and go.

THE VISCERAL TRUTH

When there's a hard truth that needs to be spoken, to this day I feel a quivery response inside my heart or belly or genitals or thighs. If I ignore it, I go numb. If I speak that truth, however, I feel a rush. I've noticed that even now, I speak pretty honestly all the time, but then when I hit a new layer and a deeper truth to penetrate, I have to do the dance all over again with the excitement, fear, and nausea.

When Speaking Truth, find and speak to the highest and best intentions of the other person. Once I was working with a client in a healing ceremony, and the Sacred Ones nudged me: I almost puked on her. Saliva started flooding my molars. I felt waves of nausea churning inside me. I went into all these self-mutilating thoughts; I'd battled bulimia for years and thought I'd gotten over it, but here was my old demon back again. Then all of a sudden, I got this feeling inside me. Maybe it wasn't about me at all; maybe this was a signal I was picking up from my client. *Should I say something to this woman or not?* I didn't know her well and might offend her. Then I heard a voice inside me say very clearly: *Ask her.* I screamed silently at the Sacred Ones, *You want me to say that? Are you fucking kidding me?* I finally asked her, "Have you ever heard of bulimia?" She did in fact have that problem. We tracked the experience that set her up for bulimia. We talked and cried into first light of the next day. Her knot of anxiety, tension, and self-loathing dissolved.

Honesty isn't the same as full-on disclosure. If I ask you a question that's deeply personal, "I prefer not to answer that" or "I'm not going there with you" is a Truth Speaker's perfectly reasonable response. It's honest while allowing you to refrain from revealing your deep and tender parts to just anybody.

Speaking Truth to a romantic partner is a great challenge. Each of us brings our individual baggage, our conditioning, our different personalities to the relationship. We have really weird rules around love. For example, there's a lot of blahblah about unconditional love. That's not what I see most of the time. I see: *I love you, you love me; therefore, you have to jump through the if-you-love-me hoops I've devised.* Changing that takes a lot of discernment on both sides to find the truth in the relationship. Take the challenge of Speaking Truth to your beloved: Can you have a conversation that disobeys these old rules? Can you go through the act of sex completely unshielded? How about for one minute and expand from there? Can you make Truth Speaking an exaltation, an intermingling of the energies of love and passion without making each other dive through the if-you-love-me hoops?

Speaking Truth about the things that are the most precious to you can be just as difficult as speaking a difficult truth. It can be as hard to say, "I really appreciate you for doing that" as to say, "What you did isn't okay. Here's what I need you to do instead."

One day I was sitting in ceremony, praying for help on speaking more effectively to my students. I wasn't quite sure what I was reaching for. The message I received was that it was time to start speaking about Spirit and helping others connect to theirs. I went instantly to war with that. At that point, I only knew how to connect with my own Spirit. It wasn't something I could bear to share because it was so precious. This put me in a personal quandary. I'd been praying and calling to the Sacred Ones for such a long time. When they finally connected with me,

I didn't like what they said. I was terrified of being grouped in with all those New Age whackaberries. I wouldn't do what the Sacred Ones suggested. They withdrew.

I had to ask myself: *What is more important to me, being loyal to my fear or doing what keeps me connected to the Sacred Ones?* My desire for that connection won out, but I had to use my fear to hone speaking in an authentic way. I honored the fear, listened to it, but wouldn't obey it. At the roots of my fear was something worth paying attention to: I wanted to be authentic. I didn't want to be a hypocrite like the New Agers who spoke about Spirit without ever being connected to it; that only drove people farther from Spirit. I would either have to be connected to my Heart or Spirit when I spoke or be reaching for that connection as I spoke. Then it would be authentic and true.

When I finally got up the courage to talk to a group of my students about connecting to Spirit, I fumbled through my talk painfully. I told them about my desire to heal others, the mission I call Mending the Hoop of the People, and how I've dedicated my entire life to it. Mending includes not only teaching but healing. I'm a really private person, and this Soul Pledge is deeply personal. Yet I realized that I couldn't accomplish my mission if I didn't talk about it, so I had to choose to make the personal be public. I was very leery about how my students would respond: *What did she just say?* Amazingly, they didn't run for the exits or exchange worried glances; they *got* it.

Afterward several came up to me and told me, "I have connected to my Spirit." I felt relieved, grateful, scared. Could I do it again? Was I delusional? Was I just a people pleaser? But I could hear my students' words resonating off my truth shield, the energetic gong inside me that could discern lies from truth. When someone Spoke Truth, I heard a beautiful resonant sound; lies sounded harsh and clunky. I could see their wisdom shining out of their eyes. We'd Spoken Truth to each other. I began to speak about connecting to Spirit more and more. Now I'm reaching for what I yearn for and speaking it; it's really risky and exciting.

SPEAKING TRUTH IF YOU'VE BEEN ABUSED

When I was younger, it was really difficult to speak about my sexual abuse and the raw mass of feelings it had left in its wake. Just about everything hurt my feelings, and whenever I tried to speak about what had happened to me, even the faintest whisper of wind going past that rawness would hurt. I felt completely invalid. I couldn't speak about what hurt me until I found professionals who really understood what I was going through. People who have been abused need a therapist, period— a competent, professional navigator to take them through the memories and feelings, the blanks and brainwashing and suicide triggers. My therapist encouraged me to speak about it to drain the backlog of hurt. My hurt often came out as blame directed toward the listener, myself, or my abusers because it was so hard to communicate, and this made it difficult for those around me to listen. It was very important for me to recognize that I wasn't responsible for the abuse, and to put the blame where it belonged. Then I needed to recognize that my healing was my responsibility. Speaking these truths about the abuse was an essential and necessary step in that healing.

Whenever I work with people who have been abused, I require them to work with a competent therapist who specializes in abuse. Being in therapy and doing Yoga is an excellent combination. I tell them that there will be a time when they will blame everyone and everything. After being silenced for so long, it's a useful phase to be able to point your finger and say, "You hurt me." To say, "This was his sickness, not mine," is a really important step. But then you must move on and take responsibility for your healing. Reaching out to the professionals who can help you is not only essential, but the absolutely most compassionate thing you can do for yourself. You cannot do it alone; disobey the dictates of abuse that tell you that you must. Isolation is part of the abuse conditioning. This is where you must reach out.

SPOTTING THE LAND MINES THAT SABOTAGE TRUTH SPEAKING

Whenever you Speak Truth to someone else, you're making an energetic connection; you need to be responsible for your part of the communication, but for no more. I still stumble with this but have figured out some of the ways my own biases can damage the process. Do any of these sound familiar?

For example, as a problem solver, I'm fairly fearless about looking at whatever's gone wrong. I'm challenged in recognizing what's going beautifully. Keeping this balance attunes me to a bigger truth.

That side of me I call Firefighter swings into crisis mode and gets the job done. I'm great in a crisis. I'm used to gathering info, making a coherent story, making decisions, and acting on them pronto. As a healer, that's what I do. When your house is burning down, you want Firefighter on call. But she's not so great in ordinary living. Without meaning to, I can shift into crisis mode when it's not appropriate. In my well-intentioned efforts to help, I might overprotect someone else without asking whether it's what he wants or needs.

The side of me I call Sacrificial Whore can also sabotage communication and my own needs. In my work, I want to send out Beauty and healing. However, my sense of mission can make me so desperate to do good in the world that I sacrifice time for myself. For example, in our teacher training courses, my teaching team and I use the sanctity of our personal Yoga practice together to brainstorm how to work with a student's challenge or injury. This is a noble endeavor, but the wrong time and place. Our practice time is for us, and the teaching time is for our students. We remind each other to refocus by Speaking Truth in a humorous way. This reinforces our teachings of nurturing our own body *and* Spirit.

Yes, you need to open your heart, but you have to have the support and wisdom of your brain and gut—the whole council of your being—rather than just following whichever voice happens to be really loud. Part of Truth Speaking is taking that moment to check in with your internal council. When you're in a hot, reactive moment, instead of responding in fear or anger, take a few breaths, straighten your spine, and ask the internal questions: *What is my truth right now? What can I say to help this moment of conflict come to resolution?* If you're a parent furious at a kid who comes home high, your initial impulse might be to rage, "Get out of my house! I don't want you to come home stoned!" But a moment of reflection might yield a more compassionate response: "I'm worried. I want you to be healthy. Let's talk about how we can make that happen."

My personal switchboard is hooked up so that my first response is rage. Not anger: *rage*—the kind that could light the planet. One of my earliest lessons was that if I loved anything or anyone, the best thing I could do was get it away from me before it got hurt or killed. I come from a place of rage *because* I care and I'm frightened. I might be hurt, worried, concerned—and it just looks like I'm pissed. I'm learning to breathe and feel for the truth under my first reaction.

I'm also working to break an even subtler pattern. It used to be that when I got into a verbal argument with someone, if it got hot and heavy, I knew how to sit steady through it. But if the other person became disrespectful to me, I felt he no longer had the right or privilege to know my feelings. Unconsciously, I'd start withholding my feelings—not just from him, but sometimes even from myself. The result was that I wasn't using all the information available to me to make wise choices. Now my challenge is to check in and ask, *What am I withholding, and can I speak it?* Sometimes there's so much tumultuous feeling in me that it's like a wave. I've got to sort through it before I can respond. I have to track it back.

In a hot moment, it's difficult to go inside and chat with your internal council, but that's exactly what you need to do. Stop, get your feet active, and get rooted through your legs. Then take a few deep breaths and feel around inside for your heart—you'll have a better chance of responding from your heart rather than just reacting.

A final land mine that can blow up communication is disconnection. We've all had those moments when we go on autopilot, when we seem to be listening but we're really just brain-dead. Tune in to the words you repeat a lot when you're in conversation with someone else; typical ones are *I see, you know, yeah, um,* and *uh-huh.* Are you using these words to keep the conversation flowing or as verbal placeholders while your mind travels elsewhere? Breathe and track the moments when you're disconnecting. It's part of the awakening process of Truth Speaking.

PHYSICAL FOCUS:
POSES TO STRENGTHEN AND OPEN THE HEART

Rachel, one of my students, had Bell's palsy, which had frozen part of her face. The nerves there were dead, unfeeling. The paralysis was more widespread than it appeared; Rachel had learned to bottle up her feelings and shield her heart. She told me, "I have these inconvenient emotions." "Inconvenient for whom?" I asked. For everyone around her, apparently. Through our work on the mat, Rachel began to cry and let loose, and I gave her the space to feel safe as she did it. This emotional cardio started to thaw her inside and out, catalyzing a huge shift inside her as those so-called inconvenient emotions began to surface. As she learned to stay with them, Rachel began to realize that she had to speak the truth to a lot of people who wouldn't be particularly pleased to hear it. The more she spoke her truth, the more nerve response began to return in her face. Getting in touch with her feelings literally enabled her to feel.

When you're becoming a Truth Speaker, specific poses can help you focus inside, strengthen, and begin opening the heart, and then muster the fire and courage to speak. The following poses work well for this. I also like to do Handstand (see page 34) to turn the world upside down. When you go upside down, you not only bring oxygen to your brain, but you treat yourself to some risk and exhilaration, which is just what speaking the truth is like. When you have that excitement of going upside down, it's just the energy you need. *Hey, yeah! I did a handstand! Now I can handle my boss/partner/empty page for school.* Handstand helps you break through like nothing else.

UJJAYI BREATHING

Ujjayi breathing is the easiest way to help you focus inside. It will strengthen your quality of attention and cue you to stretch your breath to its fullest capacity. Ujjayi brightens the bioenergetic field (your aura) almost immediately. It's a cleansing breath that heats up the body, stimulates the parasympathetic response in the nervous system (which quiets the mind), and brings on the relaxation response. Ujjayi breath opens your throat, which is where your fifth chakra is located—the place from which you express yourself. Bringing the aliveness of your breath over your vocal cords will help open them so you can open yourself to Truth Speaking.

Whisper "hello" to feel where and how your breath travels over the vocal cords in the back of the throat. With your mouth open, inhale, drawing breath through the mouth and over the back of the throat— making a sound similar to a sigh or whisper. Exhale air through your open mouth, moving the breath over the back of the throat—making a whisper sound. Repeat this sound with your mouth open a few times, and then continue Ujjayi with your mouth closed. (Some people have described this sound as Darth Vader breathing.) It's easier to get it on the exhale; that's a good enough win for the day. Sometimes it takes a few sessions to get Ujjayi on the inhale. Move with your Ujjayi breath, utilizing it as a tool to stay present, alert, and in feeling. Move with the intelligence of what you're feeling. Stay conscious! It's way more fun.

CORE-STRENGTHENING POSES

You also need to have the guts (literally) and support for your heart to do Truth Speaking. The core strengtheners Elbow to Knee, Abs with a Roll, and Frog Lifting Through (see page 59–60) help you with Truth Speaking and will strengthen your heart. Here are some other poses I recommend.

LUNGES WITH LION'S BREATH

Standing poses can teach you how to take a stance for what matters to you. When you develop and use the strength of your legs, you learn to trust that you're powerful enough to walk your life path and speak for yourself. Lunges with Lion's Breath is a terrific way of opening all your energy centers, especially those from the thighs and pelvis on up. You want to access all the power in your thighs, pelvis, and gut to tap in to your inner fire and courage. When you first want to Speak Truth, you might have this burning force inside you as you feel all the times that your voice was shut down, you were told to shut up, or your life force was suffocated. Lunges with Lion's Breath can help free up that energy so you can say what you need to say.

Come into your Lunge (see page 29). Inhale into or toward the part of your body that has the trapped energy. Exhale forcibly through a wide-open mouth. Stretch your tongue toward your chin and *roar*! Do three to five roars on each side.

CAMEL HANDS ON HEELS

Camel stimulates the thighs and pelvis, opens the heart, and frees up the throat when you let your head relax back. It's a rib opener and a back strengthener as well. Warm up for Camel by doing eight Elbow to Knee (see page 58) and eight Sun Salutations (see page 223) first.

Move into Camel (see page 30). Remain in the pose for five to eight breaths; it takes that long to get past *I hate this pose* to where the sweetness is. To move into Camel Hands on Heels, come into Camel, inhale with hands on hips, then exhale, easing your hands down one at a time onto your heels. If your neck is okay, relax your head back and telescope your ribs up; otherwise keep your head toward your chest. Stay long in the back and lift your chest to the ceiling. To transition out of the pose, put one hand at a time back on your sacrum, lift your torso upright, lift your head, and sit back on your heels.

CAMEL ON THE WALL

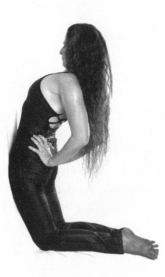

Camel on the Wall

If you have a sensitive back, you can do Camel on the Wall. Face a wall and press your thighs, pubic bone, and low ribs onto the wall. Place your hands on your sacrum, thumbs on either side of the spine and fingers curving toward your hips. Drag your low ribs up the wall, decompressing the lower back. Arch your chest up and away from the wall. Keep your chin toward your chest, shoulders down, and press your elbows toward each other.

CHEST OPENER ON THE WALL

Chester Opener on the Wall is a great way to open the heart and bring breath to it. However, it's a very inward pose because even though it opens your heart, your throat can remain closed. Stand with your right side twelve inches from a wall. Step into Warrior I (see page 62), right leg forward. Place your right hand on the wall behind your back, arm shoulder height or slightly lower if your shoulder is tight. Put your left hand on your right upper chest or over the heart. Inhale into your heart and chest. Feel your chest move under your hand. Exhale, turning your torso slightly to the left, increasing the stretch. If this pulls too intensely in the shoulders, move both feet a couple inches farther from the wall. Feel for freeing up your heart, chest, and lungs with each breath. Do four to five breaths on each side.

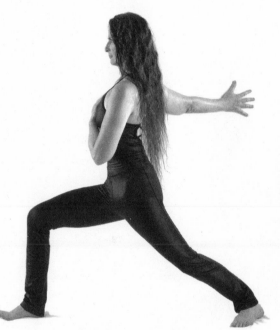

Chest Opener on the Wall

The way you speak, the way you breathe—that's some pretty primal behavior to change. Yet becoming a Truth Speaker allows you to step into your most powerful, authentic self. It's worth the effort. Take a breath, feel your heart, get conscious, and speak from your heart. It's a skill we all need to exercise.

4

THE FIERCEST MEDICINE:
A BRIEF PAUSE WHILE YOU DIE

RAIN IS A MAGICAL EVENT in the desert, unlocking all the potential that's been hiding just under the surface. If you sit still long enough, you can almost see it go green and bloom in front of your eyes, until the entire horizon is carpeted orange, gold, and blue with wildflowers. It's a beauty made vibrant by its very transience, the imminence of its death making it all the more poignant.

One day right after a shower, I sat for a while under a tree by the lower paddock. smelling the rain, my anger and fear and loneliness gnawing inside me. I was seventeen, out in the desert, training horses, trying to make my own reputation, thinking maybe I could start my own business. My heart wasn't in it, though. Why bother? I'd lived so long in suffering and despair, I didn't see any other way to be. I sat there waiting for the green to come, but for something else too, I wasn't sure what.

The clouds shifted, and a rainbow lit up the sky above me, arcing into the near distance, just over the next rise. There was the rainbow's end, I decided, just within reach. I wasn't looking for the legendary pot of gold, but something good, something magical. I knew that legends started for a reason, some small grain of truth, and that there must be something there for me.

I saddled up Squirrel—he was a very fast thoroughbred who never tired—and went chasing straight after the end of that rainbow. I had it in my mind that the end of the rainbow was a gateway into the realm of fairies, a magical world within the world. I could see exactly where the rainbow ended. If I could just reach it: escape. I galloped toward it; it disappeared. Oh, over there! I thundered toward it again—gone. What I didn't know was that rainbows can jump depending on your perspective. Again and again it dodged me. And the farther it moved, the more I leaned into Squirrel's neck and dug in my heels and the more I could feel the last spark of hope in me dwindle, until finally the hope flickered out in the desert rain. I reined my horse in. That magical gateway, the end of the rainbow, was still in front of me, but to my mind the magic was irrevocably rejecting me because I was such an incredibly foul and poisonous creature.

That, I decided, was my last attempt at life. I was really, really done. My life was futile. Time to go. Time to die.

The next day I rode out among the new flowers on a scouting expedition. It didn't take me long to find the right spot: a tall mesa above a dry arroyo layered thickly with river rock. I looked out around me among the Joshua trees; I could see for miles. I stared down over the lip of the cliff, over thirty or forty feet high, tall enough to make death a sure thing. Everywhere below, rocks jutted up menacingly. This was the place.

I rode back to the ranch, stabled and fed the horses, and gave them a lot of water. I desperately hoped that someone would come check on them before too long, that they'd be safe from the snakes and coyotes. I loved them so much; they'd been my only true friends. Walking from paddock to paddock, I petted the horses and blew gently into their nostrils. I sent pictures to them in my mind—since that's how we talked to each other—pictures of vacant space that said: *I'm not here anymore.* Open vistas, empty paddocks. I was gone.

I scratched Squirrel's favorite itch spots. I stroked his nostrils, so soft they felt like velvet. I felt saddest of all to be leaving him. He was a coppery chestnut, bright as a buffed-up penny, with a very pretty blaze down his face. He'd been a little psycho when I bought him, not mean, just unwilling to be ridden. We hung out a lot together, and eventually he let me ride him.

I thought of all the foals I'd midwifed, the horses I'd healed. But that was all over. I knew I could no longer carry the burden of their life forces. I couldn't carry the burden of my *own* life force.

As the sun set, I headed back to the cliff alone on foot. As always, the pain of my wonky legs lanced through my body and my left foot dragged. But tonight, the pain didn't matter to me. It's only when we think we have to live with pain that it becomes suffering. I wasn't going to have to live with it much longer. Goodbye to all that. I sat down close to the edge of the cliff and stared up into the darkening sky. At first my mind chattered away about dying, the utter hopelessness of life. Then, slowly, it quieted. It was a beautiful, clear desert night. I quit thinking about anything at all as a rare peacefulness stole over me. A hundred million stars twinkled above me, and the soft air wrapped itself around me. Because I was done with everything, because I didn't care anymore, I could finally, fully, feel the preciousness of the moment, like the transient feeling when the rains came, only deeper. The night, the stars, the cliff . . . all held nothing more or less than pure beauty. For once in my life, I felt calm, serene.

Right. Now. I stood up, I ran, and I jumped off the cliff. I was flying and still watching the stars, no regrets.

I don't remember any pain from the impact. Did shock shield me from it? Did my soul step out of my body before I hit the earth? I don't know. I've imagined what it must have felt like, but I can't separate my imagination from my reality. All I know is that I was unconscious for a while; then I woke up, a little disoriented. When I realized I wasn't dead, I was fucking *furious*. I was spitting sand, wiping it out of my eyes, my hair, my nose, my ears. Sand everywhere. Sand? I looked around. I'd landed in a pile of sand that most definitely hadn't been there earlier in the day. How had that happened? There was no way in hell I could have survived hitting those rocks, and I knew for sure that the sand pile hadn't been there earlier.

Now what?

This hadn't been a cry for help; I'd been determined to end my suffering. But all I was stuck with was enormous bruises and abrasions and a killer headache. I struggled to my feet and walked slowly back to the barn, limping, growling, swearing, aching—all that pain I was going to have to keep living with. When I got back to the barn, I just threw myself down and watched the bruises purple up while I dug more sand out of my skin. I was so shocked that for some unbelievable reason I was still alive.

I now understand that the Sacred Ones did a little intervention that day. I guess they weren't ready to let me end my life. They wanted me to *start* my life, a real one, a life with purpose. At seventeen, I didn't know how or what that life would look like, but I was starting to realize that I'd been given a chance to test my courage by living.

DANCING WITH DEATH

Since my leap off that cliff, I've had lots of opportunities to witness how being close to death can be a time of terrifying clarity. Dancing with death—being with the dying, working with the energy of death, even snuggling up to it—has taught me by far the most powerful lessons about life.

In my twenties, I began training with energetic healer and medium Rosalyn Bruyere. Rosalyn is a Medicine Woman of the Hopi, Navajo, and Cree Nations, well versed in diagnosing where people's energy was dimmed. She could feel people's energetic blockages through her hands and use her own focus and energy to reopen those channels. I hoped that studying with her would channel and direct my own powers of healing and walk me into magic.

My study with Native American Medicine People has taught me that it's crucial to recognize each aspect of yourself like the facets of a gemstone and give it a place and purpose within you. That way, it won't sabotage you or come out in shocking and inappropriate ways, as can so often happen. When I understood that, I began to accept and invite other aspects into my circle as my healing partners. I drew from other traditions so that I could become a more integrated and effective healer.

My studies included teaching Yoga and running energy, an ancient practice of drawing on the forces of nature. When I run energy, I move the *prana,* or life force, through my heart and hands into another person. That person's innate intelligence deploys this energetic gift as it sees fit. I would run energy on really sick people, people near death with

AIDS and cancer. These were people at a crossroads: they were either going to get better, or they were going to die. My role was to midwife the process in whatever direction it flowed, but I didn't get that at first. I thought my mission was: save them. If I couldn't fulfill that, I thought I failed. The work was intense, so as a healer, I learned to summon the energy of Kali, the Hindu goddess of death and destruction, to help me.

Kali is one murderous bitch of a goddess. She's the one with the burning red eyes, black skin stained with blood, necklace of skulls, girdle of severed arms, and purse made from a human head. My kind of gal. (My therapist once told me, "No wonder you chose Kali as a goddess, considering your mother!") And here's the thing about Kali: she's one fierce chick, but she's also revered as a nurturing Mother Goddess. She compassionately sweeps away what needs to die so that what deserves to live can survive. When I laid hands on my patients or guided them in various Yoga poses, I'd send her energy in to hunt, stalk, and kill the mass, the lesion, whatever it was, to sweep out whatever was dead and rotting to make room for vital tissue.

My choice of Kali as a healing partner might be frowned upon by some in the Yoga world, where one of the most sacred principles is *ahimsa,* the vow of nonviolence, the pledge to do no injury to sentient beings. But I've never taken that vow; that's not how I roll. I am *so* not the turn-your-cheek person. (This is why those nice Jainists never invite me to their picnics.) So I spent a lot of time studying this Hindu goddess revered for her ability to slay demons, carry off the bodies of great warriors and animals, suck the blood of her enemies. Her fierceness was exactly what I needed in my healing work. Instead of suffocating Kali's qualities already present in me, I wanted to invite her into my circle as my healing partner. It was a good, sacred place for that ferocious person inside me.

Before I learned about Kali, I hadn't known what to do with my rage and desire for destruction born of the abuse I'd endured. I'd turned that murderous impulse on myself with all my self-destructive behavior. To my horror and shame, I'd even turned it on the horses I loved, beating on them when they disobeyed. I thought the leap off the cliff would kill the killer inside me. I was wrong. My task wasn't to kill off that part of myself; it was to understand and ally with that big energy and temper it with compassion. Kali represented one of the first aspects of female Spirit I could begin to honor.

It took me a while to realize that Kali could do so much more than merely stalk and kill. She represents not just the destructive power of death, but Ultimate Reality—what you get when you stare your own mortality in the face. She's a warrior who can help others make a Warrior's Choice to face the truth of their dying, and the truth of how they want to spend what time they have left on earth. Kali is the ultimate Truth Speaker. And there is never a more important time to Speak Truth than when you're dying.

Until Bill, a young patient in his twenties, came into my life, I didn't appreciate the sacred opportunities that come with facing death. Bill was a student of mine who had ended up in the hospital with end-stage complications from AIDS. When I came to visit, I found him swallowed up in his hospital bed, wired up to monitors, his arms laced with IVs. His face and arms were purple with lesions. He looked frail and emaciated, alone and very, very sick. One look, and I knew I wasn't going to be able to make Bill better. So what could I do for him? I felt Kali nudge me toward another equally important role of a healer: to be a Truth Speaker. I hiked my chair up next to Bill's bed and threaded my hand through the IVs so I could clasp his. "How do you feel about dying?" I asked him.

Bill burst into tears of relief. "No one's spoken the truth to me. Everyone keeps telling me I'm gonna get better."

"Well, you look like you're dying to me. How do you feel about that?" It was as if a dam had burst. Bill spilled out his nightmares about dying. He interrupted his story a few times to cough all over me, and I could feel his blood and mucus spray my face. It felt like the kiss of death—this was before people really understood what AIDS was and how it was transmitted. In that one moment, I had to face the fear of my own death; I was convinced that I'd just gotten infected with this deadly, incurable, hideous disease. It deepened our intimacy. Bill and I were Speaking Truth, looking at our own deaths together. I figured if this was the way I was going out, at least I could do something useful with my time. I just wiped the blood and spit off and continued working with Bill as best I could.

Over the next visits, I helped him place calls so he could die with his heart unburdened. Kali helped me heal Bill's spirit. I helped him puzzle through what his terrifying dreams meant to him. In one dream, Bill was on a boat on a river, racing down currents beyond his control. I talked to him about the River Styx, the mythology of facing one's death with courage and integrity. When he began to understand that he was dreaming what his soul was telling him to do to prepare for his death, his dreams became a source of guidance, not terror. In his last dream, he was facing forward in the boat, looking out ahead, at peace. Our last few hours together were sacred, authentic. Bill was fully present even as his soul withdrew from his body.

Helping Bill was a really big turning point for me. When the lesions went into his brain and he died, at first it felt like a horrendous loss—he was very young, and even though I'd worked hard to help him die with integrity, part of me had really just wanted him to live, and I'd hoped against hope that my healing work would accomplish that. So at first, I felt like I'd failed him. My heart and soul were in such pain because he was so precious to me. But then I recognized that I had a prejudice: although I'd helped Bill embrace his own death, I was still stuck in the belief that I was supposed to help him live. Because I was grieving the loss of someone so dear, I failed to recognize and honor the great service I had done for him. Bill and I had given each other great gifts.

BEAUTY REPORTS

I started working with my other dying patients as I had with Bill. I abandoned my bias that I was there to save them and started asking them, "What do you care most about *right now*? What can I do to make your passage through this gateway have the most integrity possible? How can I make you proud of your death?" Maybe they needed help making that phone call so they could say a final goodbye to someone they loved— or to make peace with someone they hated. Maybe they just wanted someone to give them their medication or rub their feet. I discovered that those final months, weeks, days, minutes could be incredibly precious and vital—as long as people Spoke Truth, faced up to their rackets and delusions, and focused on what really mattered to them. We talked about regrets—how they would have spent their lives if they only had more time—but more importantly, we focused on how they could live their last moments authentically. My assignment to them was to gather Beauty Reports to share when I came over to visit. I asked them to step out of their suffering, look around, and find something that touched their heart in Beauty.

I learned the full power of Beauty Reports from Diane, a lovely woman whose body was slowly destructing because of cancer. She'd decided to spend her final days at home, and I visited her there regularly, helping her with her breathing, which was difficult with her lungs stiffened with tumors. She lay there choking and gagging as I ran energy on her, willing her bronchial tubes to expand and bring her more precious oxygen. She struggled beneath my hands.

I described to her the stone hoodoos I'd seen in Utah, majestically twisting, crazy spires of rock that seem to defy gravity as they reach heavenward. "How do you think they were shaped?" I asked her. "They were shaped by the wind. That's how you need to breathe with these tumors. You just need to breathe like the wind shaping the stone, breath shaping bone." As I helped Diane focus on drawing in air around the blockages in her lungs, the wind swirling around the tumors, sculpting them but not conflicting with them, her breathing would calm, and her body would grow more peaceful.

Together Diane and I figured out how to surrender to other struggles too. As her pain increased and standing became more difficult, her life shrunk to her bed where she lay tethered to various life support machines. It became our task to bring the world to her. "What's the Beauty Report today?" I'd ask her. "What did you see today that had Beauty?"

Her young son's smile. The flowers outside the window. Even the noisy teenagers next door whose antics sometimes disturbed her rest. Diane found Beauty in them all. We made a point of exchanging our Beauty Reports at every meeting, telling each other what mattered most at that very moment. She was amazing—so close to death, yet she'd lie there and insist, "I have a brilliant life." She did have one regret, a goal she hadn't fulfilled. An ardent student of Buddhism, she'd wanted to be a bodhisattva, a being bound for enlightenment whose wisdom is an inspiration to others. When I told a Buddhist friend about her, he smiled with delight. "But she *is* a bodhisattva! She's laying there dying and yet she's expressing concern for others." I shared his insight with Diane, who took great joy in his observation.

Finally, though, it was clear that it was time for Diane's body to surrender; she'd had enough of fighting her disease, enough of the hideous pain racking her body. But she was hesitant to give up the struggle. "What do you need to accomplish before you die?" I asked her.

"I can't go," she told me. "I'm tied down by the people I love." Dying would mean abandoning her beloved husband and young son, a prospect too heartbreaking to contemplate. Yet it was too painful to stay.

"Diane, you need to use our love for you as your wings," I told her. "Not to tie you down, but to ride on out. There's no coming back for you, Diane. It's time to ride out." Diane sank back, her body visibly relaxing. This made sense to her. She'd needed permission and a path to depart. Now she had both. She could face death using her great love for family and friends to accomplish the transformation into Spirit. Diane slid into a coma and a few days later died, at peace with herself and at peace with death.

SHAMAN'S DEATH

After helping so many others deal with dying bodies and souls, I realized that I needed to summon Kali once again to help me in my own life. By this time, I'd done a lot of therapy to come to grips with all the sexual and emotional abuse I'd suffered. Inside me was a very wounded little girl who needed rescuing. I'd spent a lot of time in therapy trying to get that little girl to speak to me. She remained a silent ball of shame, damage, rage. It was time to confront this pocket of rot that she embodied. I found some Native American Medicine People willing to guide me through a sacred ceremony called Shaman's Death, part of which would take place in a sweat lodge. There I would greet this little girl and Speak Truth with her. We would heal each other.

On the appointed day, I lifted up a corner of the heavy blankets covering the willow frame, got down on my hands and knees, and crawled inside the sweat lodge. Steam rose up as the Fire Keeper poured more water on the glowing coals in the center of the sweat lodge. Three of us sat cross-legged in a circle around it. The thick air was suffocating, and sweat poured off my skin. Sometimes I had to bury my nose in the dirt to keep from passing out. As the ceremony proceeded, the Medicine People encouraged me to bring this little girl inside of me forward for the final healing, but she couldn't do it. This tiny, scraggly, broken scrap of a thing with the long hair and sad eyes was beyond saving. I knew it then: she had to die. She'd absorbed so much abuse that it had fatally poisoned her. We were both heartbroken; I wanted so badly to bring her into the light, but she wanted death, begged for it. I'd spent so much time and energy trying fruitlessly to heal a part of myself. Now it was time to kill it off so that I could move ahead with my life. I could feel the energy of Kali pushing me forward: *life from death.*

In ceremony, guided by my wise elders, I pictured that wounded little girl in front of me holding all the damage from the abuse she suffered. She folded herself around the damage like an oyster encapsulates granules of sand. In a visionary way, I drew a sharp knife and disemboweled her, so that the rot and disease could be freed from her little body. I took her in my arms and buried her in a peaceful meadow where I used to hang out with the horses. I let the virulent, pustulant, evil energy that had been encapsulated inside her pour out into Mother Earth, turn into fertilizer for the grass. Life from death. Goodness from evil.

When I crawled back out of the sweat lodge, I pulled the clear, cool air into my lungs and cried for the little girl I'd killed. I cried for the sadness and the sweetness and the joy and the hope of it all. She'd given her life so that I could truly live—*if* I chose to. Once again, the Sacred Ones were showing me that I must actively choose life.

SPIRITUAL FOCUS:
THE FIERCEST MEDICINE

Facing your death is truly the fiercest medicine. My commitment to life, and my life's work, come from these powerful lessons I've learned about death—my leap off the cliff, understanding Kali's role in my life, working with dying patients, and the Shaman's Death ceremony. It's amazing what a little dying can do for you. When I train students who want to teach Forrest Yoga, I want them to discard whatever is holding them back. Then they can discover what matters most to them and bring that forth as they learn to become healers and Yoga teachers. In Kali fashion, I created a ceremony that would give them the chance to explore what piercing the boundary between life and death has to offer. I call it the Death Meditation.

The Death Meditation is an intense process in which I guide people through their last day on earth, counting down the hours, the minutes. Far beyond some morbid exercise, this is a very keen blade that cuts through the mental chatter and detritus that fill up our heads—*I can't reach for what I want because of this, or that, or whatever.* It's hard to discover what you really want if you're full of all this useless poison and these self-mutilating thoughts. The Death Meditation gets you focusing with diamond-sharp clarity on what matters. Because all facades, delusions, rackets, and life-sucking trivia pale when you face your impending death.

The Buddha said, "If you want to know what your future will be like, then look at your life right now." I see life as a huge tree, with many different colored leaves. Each leaf of the tree must eventually fall and die, turning into compost to feed the roots of this great tree of life. The Death Meditation is an opportunity to check out what's hanging onto your tree of life. Are there a few things that are ready to die and become compost to feed your tree, or are they still sucking aliveness from it? Death must occur to make room for the new leaves and flowers.

We have to be willing to let the part within us that needs to die go through that same cycle. It's all about shattering and reforming, shattering and reforming. We have to make room to grow. Otherwise, all that crap just accumulates and we get backed up with psychic constipation. Whatever it is that drags and dims your life force has to die. Whatever you cannot transform, you must either form a new relationship with or shed. That's my bottom line: evolve or die.

The Death Meditation will bring you face to face with what you need to let go and how you need to move ahead. What needs to fall away so you can fulfill your life's purpose? If you let yourself embrace the process, which is a kind of vision quest—the search for a new way to live your life—you'll walk in a different way afterward, and you can begin to

build a support system for the new way you choose to live. It'll be easier for you to let stuff go; when you know what you're here for, you're not
going to want to waste your life force on petty things.

I introduce the Death Meditation at the midpoint in my three-week-
long teacher training. In order to get my students to live and teach
authentically, I begin the Yoga ceremony by calling in the powers, attributes, and protection of the Four Directions: East, South, West, and
North. I direct each person to set his or her intent for the day, which
aligns them for their meditation and intense daily Yoga practice. This
is how they discover the voice of their own Spirit, which guides them
through their right life path. The work we do together is pretty fierce.
We spend the first few days in teardown, digging into the past so we can
get down to the foundation and make sure it's solid before we rebuild.
It's a very emotional time, lots of crying and shaking and releasing. By
day eleven, everyone has pretty much degenerated into a four-year-old.
They need to shed all the old crap and find out what's up ahead.

Another name for my Death Meditation is the Shaman's Death. I
know that this incredible, painful ceremony of dragging my students
through their own deaths will leave them cleansed from the parasitic
and dulling behaviors and energies that keep them from living their
brilliant, authentic selves. Taking them through the Death Meditation
ceremony is a great act of compassion, although it is painful. I tell my
trainees, "You've been making the same mistakes for eleven days. After
the Death Meditation, you have to make new mistakes."

I've placed the Death Meditation at this point in the book because
I want you to bring clarity to your life's priorities just as my students
do. Right now, find out what you are honestly ready to let go of in your
life, and what you most yearn to go after. This knowledge will galvanize
you for the work that comes in the following chapters. You'll be ready to
make your own new mistakes and discoveries as you move toward your
right life.

People are Velcroed to their known and familiar miseries. Just at the
moment they're faced with the wide-open space of the unknown, they
start grabbing at their old paradigm because it's familiar and not scary.
I created the Death Meditation to help you launch yourself off the cliff
into the unknown. You've finally stripped off the leashes and tethers—

now jump, before you reattach! Refuse to travel the old neurological pathways. Create new ones and travel them over and over and over. This is your quantum leap! Go!

So now it's time for you to die. Today. At this very moment. I'm going to guide you through your own Death Meditation as you experience your last day on earth. Together we'll count down the hours, the minutes, the seconds, your final precious moments on earth. As your life force dims, you'll ponder important questions you may have avoided your entire life.

Here's how this will go: Get a notebook, pen, and tissues and find a comfortable place to sit where you won't be disturbed for at least an hour. As you read each paragraph below, close your eyes, breathe, and take the time to absorb what it means and to allow yourself to react to it. Whatever comes up for you, write it down. You might have a physical reaction: shaking, trembling, a deep chill, numbness. Take notes on how your body feels. If a big emotional thing comes up, take the time to experience it. Tears? Fear? Shame? Confusion? Don't just shut down with it. There's no clock ticking here; move at your own pace. Your notes will be there for you to reflect on later, so stay in each moment. Keep breathing, and remain compassionate toward yourself. This is hard, brave work you're doing.

The more you put into this, the more you'll get out of it. If you sit and resist what I've written, what I'm saying, you'll just get pissy. And that's a waste of time. Go for this 100 percent, and you'll get a lot out of it. When I sat staring up at the stars before my leap off the cliff, I was able to experience peace for the first time in my life because something in me had allowed me to let go of all the chatter and simply surrender to the process. I was willing to let go of absolutely everything. Now I'm asking you to do the same: surrender to the process and face Death.

Let's begin.

THE DEATH MEDITATION

I recommend you begin this exercise in the early evening, so the fading light and the cooling air help create the correct atmosphere.

Write at the top of your paper, *Death Meditation.*

Now close your eyes. Have your writing materials open in front of you as you get your breathing very deep. Get your core wide open and spacious. Feel your breath moving through your lungs, feel your own heart beating, feel your blood moving through your veins, these rivers of life moving through you.

Now consider: if you knew that in twelve hours, you would be dead, what would you do now, for these last twelve hours of your life? Without a doubt, no matter what you did—run away, kick and scream, curse me or the heavens—it wouldn't matter because you'd still be dead before morning. No escape. Get a feel for that. This is your last little bit of life. You won't even get to see another sunrise. Breathe that in, feel the truth of that. All the plans, all the things you were waiting to do in the future: they're gone. Maybe you were planning on becoming a teacher or a pilot or a lawyer or a Yoga teacher. Maybe you wanted a mate or children. Maybe when you were finally healed enough you were going to allow yourself to love. But now it's too late for all that. Feel that. In the midst of that feeling, taste how precious each moment now becomes because you have so few of them left. Take a very deep breath and savor it fully. This is one of your last breaths.

Now get ready to ask yourself some questions.

1 Feel the Death of your hopes and dreams. Everything you were getting ready for. As you sit here feeling that Death, that loss, what are your regrets? All the ways you were going to live your life, all the dreams you were waiting to live. . . . What were the promises that you made to yourself or your loved ones that you can no longer keep because your time is over? Perhaps you told yourself you'd start caring for yourself in a kind and sane way someday in the future; well, now you don't have a future. Let yourself fully feel your loss. *Write down your regrets.*

Think about all the feelings you normally keep shut away because you have to function; well, there's nothing left to function for anymore. Be brave enough to feel fully now without any guard because these are the last few feelings you get to have. Take another deep breath, feeling your regrets, your loss. Feel just how precious your life is. Now you only have eleven hours and fifty minutes left to live.

2 What are your unfinished communications? What did you want to say or write to your loved ones? To the people who touched your heart . . . or who broke it? What are the communications you need to complete before you die? To those who hurt you, those you hate, those you love? *Write down everything you wished you could say to those people. Be 100 percent honest.*

Stay connected to your breath, to the reality of your Death coming closer. As you feel your impending Death looming over you, ask yourself: *What am I still withholding? What's behind my inhibitions? Am I waiting for the right time to feel fully or express myself fully? Why?* Think about all the rules that have kept you inhibited from doing what your Spirit yearns for—and now it's too late. Your time is up. *Write down what you're holding back.*

3 As you feel your impending Death coming closer—feel that coolness of Death coming closer—realize there is really no escape from your Death. Take a breath, and allow yourself to savor the pain because it means you are still alive. As you're feeling the dread coolness of Death, ask yourself: *What am I still imprisoned by? Answer honestly.*

Take a deep breath, savor that your lungs and heart still work. Feel, for maybe the first time, how your breath sparkles through you, something you never took the time to notice before. Feel just how precious these last breaths are . . . these last breaths of life.

4 As you feel your Death begin to strip away your delusions of immortality and comfortable numbness, ask: *What have I been lying to myself about? What are all the ways I've sabotaged myself?* As your Death strips away the lies, can you finally be completely honest with yourself for these last few hours of your life? Check in, see if one of your lies is about how you need your lies. What can you finally be honest with yourself about? *Write down what you've been lying to yourself about and all the ways you've sabotaged yourself.*

If not now, you don't have any other when. Now is all you have. As you feel your Death touch and chill your skin, can you finally recognize what you have in your life that should have died long ago?

5 Recall the dead leaves of the tree that need to fall off and turn to compost to feed its roots. What in *your* life needs to break off and

die in order for you to live freely? An eating disorder, abuse, your illness, your pain, or a bad relationship? Which things have been eating your life force like a parasite? Are you going to continue to feed
these parasitic energies up until your last breath? *What in your life
needs to break off and die so you can live freely for your last few hours?*

Feel Death coming closer . . . coming right up to your face. Feel that
coolness of Death permeating your skin, chilling it bone deep, slowing your blood and organs. Feel this unstoppable presence of Death
coming into you. Take another breath; it's one of your last . . . treasure
it. As the cold invades your extremities, feel that loss of sensitivity in
your fingers and toes, your hands and feet as your life force fades.

Now, what do you say to your loved ones, knowing that you are
not going to see them after sunrise? *What are you going to say to
them? Write down your last words to those you love.*

Take another breath. The air is getting heavier and it's harder to
pull into your lungs; the oxygen isn't moving much. Take a breath
while you still can.

Feel Death seeping through your core, slowing your blood and
heart, turning your lungs flaccid and increasingly useless. What
could you do to prepare for Death in these last few hours? What
steps could you take to have a Death with integrity, a noble Death? If
you can't have a life, what will you do in these few remaining hours
to at least have a Death that you can be proud of? *Write it down.*

Now your adrenal glands are pumping frantically. You feel your
heart; it's actually starting to beat faster . . . it's racing desperately . . .
beating faster like a trapped bird as Death closes in on you. Your vision starts to darken as you grow even colder.

6 Has it become clear to you, finally, what you really love? As Death
strips away your veils, what matters most to you? *Write it down.*

7 Feel your heart abandon its frantic efforts, slowing once more, struggling to beat. Feel Death fill every last cell and permeate your brain,
extinguishing your final thoughts on earth. Feel Death come over
your heart . . . and your heart stops . . . . At this moment, when your
vital forces are stopped, can you make a choice? Can you make a
Warrior's Choice to choose the life you most deeply desire? *Make*

that choice. Feel Death's power. Now use the power of your inevitable Death to drag out all that you are ready to let die. Feel Death's cold fingers dragging and scraping all of the scar tissue, pain, betrayal, and debris out of you, through your lungs, heart, back. Feel the rest of your Death moving through you, pulling with it the remaining garbage that needs to turn into compost. Let Death take out what you are ready to be free of.

Now, draw in a fresh breath, a breath that sparkles—the first after your return from Death, and use it to breathe out all of the foul thinking that fed that debris.

Everything that kept you from living the life that you want, that you desire, that is what your Spirit yearns for, breathe it out. Now take another breath. Fill those places that so desperately want to live with this new life force. Put breath in there. Know that Death is your ally.

Breathe out your Death. Breathe in this new life force. Sparkle up.

8 Breathe that new life back into your heart. Breathe that new life back into your lungs. Breathe that new life back into your blood and get it moving again. Feel your body slowly warming from your core outward, radiating into your arms and legs, life-giving blood warming you down to your fingers and toes. Feel yourself moving in the direction of what quickens your blood. Living your life as your Spirit desires. Living the life that quickens your blood. What are the dreams that you are willing to invest your life in now? *Write them down.*

Keep breathing as you write so you add the aliveness of your breath to your purpose, vision, and dreams, knowing they are worthy of your life force. Know the truth of this: You don't know when Death will visit you again. You don't have a moment to waste anymore. Take another breath. Now that you know what really matters to you, can you live it?

9 Keeping your realizations of the Death Meditation close to you, what reminders do you need to keep steady with yourself when your addictions and old behaviors call to you? What are you going to do instead to honor your new life, this life that is so precious? *Write down the reminders that will keep you aligned with the purpose you've just committed to fulfilling.*

Take a deep breath, washing that sparkling energy of your Spirit into those areas that Death cleansed out. Welcome your Spirit home into your body fully. You have a tremendous amount of heart and courage. Use it to move past whatever held you back and imprisoned you—commit yourself to living the life your Spirit yearns for.

Take this new commitment into your next sunrise and every sunrise.

The notes you've taken during the Death Meditation are the blueprint for your new life. Keep them close and reread them often; they will help you live the life your heart and soul most desire. In doing so, you will be a gift to the world. You have met what is Sacred in you; you have moved out what is Not! Namaste.

5

CHOOSING LIFE:
SETTING YOUR INTENT

I'D MANAGED TO jump off a cliff and not die. Instead, I'd chosen life. But it took me a while to realize that that was what I was doing. That fateful night as I struggled to my feet at the bottom of the dry, dead riverbed and hobbled slowly back to the stables, my legs in more pain than ever, all I knew was that I'd failed at death—and that it was time to slam some doors in my life.

I needed to leave the desert for good. My animals and I were malnourished from our time there. I was exhausted from all the backbreaking labor, the starvation, the guilt over stealing from the horses' supplies to feed myself. I'd learned quite a lot about training, not to mention from my trial by fire as a horse healer and midwife out there virtually alone. I decided to go back to Mike Nielsen and his hunters and jumpers. His training barn was a place where my animals and I could nurse ourselves back to health.

So there I was again in the horse show world, grooming the horses, cleaning the stalls and tack, braiding manes. Hard work and harder partying. Out in the desert, my life had been pretty solitary: no one besides the horses and coyotes to get high with. But back at the barn, once the work was done, I was right back to the nonstop drinking, smoking, and drugging. If someone won a class at a show, we'd all get taken out for drinks. If someone showed up with a bottle, we'd all drain it. And then I'd have to drag myself awake at three in the morning, hungover as all hell, to get everything pristine by the time the trainers and clients turned up.

I started practicing Yoga again. No matter how exhausted or buzzed or hungover I was from the booze, weed, pills, and cigarettes, I kept coming back to the mat. I didn't know what, I didn't know how, but the Yoga was awakening something inside me.

At around the same time, I'd heard about a Yoga teacher training retreat, a super intense, month-long course at Rancho Rio Caliente near Guadalajara, Mexico. I liked the sound of the challenge and knew it would pull me out of the show world, which I was starting to admit would end in a slow march to death. Then again, if I went, I'd have to go cold turkey and make it through a whole month without drugs, cigarettes, alcohol, or meat. The retreat cost five hundred fifty dollars, way more than I had. And I'd have to give up the animals I'd loved and lived with for so long. I was torn: stay or leave. Keep striving in the horse world or make a quantum leap toward something else that was calling me but I didn't understand at all.

In the end I figured I'd already failed at death, so I better try jumping into life, an act that required a hell of a lot more courage and faith, although I didn't even know that word. I decided to do the Yoga teacher training. I sold off my beloved Squirrel, gave most of the money to my brother so he could go to school and have his own chance at life, and used the rest to enroll in the course and buy a one-way third-class train ticket to Guadalajara.

Very few precise dates have survived the hazy curtain of all my addictions, but October 5, 1975, is one I know for sure. I caught the train to Guadalajara on that day and went dry, cold turkey. I was eighteen years old.

With my typical flare for planning, I hopped on board with no food, water, or money for a three-day trip, which meant unwitting fasting and dehydration. (I'm not sure I even knew that the trip would take three days.) But it was also a seriously magical trip because I did something really strange for me: I made two friends. Understand: I was a really mean kid. I wouldn't bark; I'd just bite. I'd perfected an attitude so effectively abrasive it kept people far, far away. And still, somehow, on the train I made two friends. There was Lupe, a Mexican woman going back home, and "the Blond," an All-American, voted-most-popular, straight-toothed athlete whom I normally never would have even spoken to.

The Blond—I don't know his real name—happened to be sitting near me when I had a seizure—the same kind of blackout followed by a blinding headache I'd been having for years. He stood guard over me during the episode and picked me off the floor afterward. "You've got epilepsy," he told me. "Fuck off!" I snapped back. He shrugged, but kept coming back to make his case. Finally I had to agree that there actually was something strange about these blackouts; my brain always felt storm-damaged afterwards, like lightning bolts had run through my head and burnt out the neurons. Now, thanks to the Blond, my symptoms all made sense. With that diagnosis, he'd given me a small piece of the puzzle of myself.

Lupe took care of me once we arrived in Guadalajara. Getting off the train, fried from the epileptic fit and the fasting, I realized I had no idea how to get to the retreat center. Lupe took charge. She put me in a taxi, spoke to the driver, paid him, and told me what to look for when I got out. It was night when I got to the retreat. I wandered around and somehow ended up in a bed. I'd arrived.

My Yoga teacher training at Rancho Rio Caliente was the most intense month of my life to date, especially because I was both feeling so alive *and* going through such radical detox in the middle of it all. One day while sitting in class, the teacher droned on about the sutras, the sacred commentaries of dead men like the Buddha and Patanjali. (I'd never once heard any lecture about any of the wise women of Yoga.) As I settled down deeply into lotus, I was both scared and amused to watch vines climb up through the floor, slowly wind around my shins, creep around my torso, and pierce my skin with their sharp thorns. I didn't flinch as snakes and hairy bird-sized tarantulas poured over my crossed legs and into my lap. In the throes of going cold turkey and surviving the shakes, shivers, and hallucinations of the DTs, it was an unusual way to build self-esteem, but I figured if I could sit still and simply watch while all this weirdness was crawling over me, maybe I was cut out for this Yoga thing after all. That was the most powerful lecture on the sutras I've ever had. It could also be why I never lecture on the sutras.

Every day I felt a little bit more of the poison seeping out of my system as I detoxed. One day I was in another trainee's room, sitting on her bed while she got ready so we could go to class. I looked down and saw a little white scorpion, maybe an inch long, crawling between my fingers. The DTs, working their hallucinatory magic again, I figured. *Look at how good I've gotten,* I thought to myself. *It's just one little bug instead of a whole stampede.* My friend looked over at me, saw the scorpion, and screamed. I was totally flummoxed. My first thought was, *What are you doing in my personal delusion?* It was a collision of two worlds. I moved my hand away from the scorpion, just to satisfy her. Then realized: holy shit—that was a real scorpion!

Our Yoga teachers had us teach a class on the last day. The teacher training program was sharing Rancho Rio Caliente with a weight-loss program, a retreat with structured meals and exercise. I decided to teach them a course I created myself, even though I was terrified because my mother and brother were also grossly overweight. It was another cliff jump for me—could I face my terror of these women and con them into letting me give them a free Yoga class?

I learned more from working with those women for four hours than in my entire teacher training. But first I had to get over my revulsion so I could put my hands on them and try not to throw up in their hair. The obese women had the same fear of failure and body inhibitions that I did. "I can't," I'd hear when I introduced the most basic poses. "I'm gonna fail if I try and I'll hate myself even more. Why am I such a disgusting slob?" I wanted to get these women out of self-loathing, so I taught them to look at the poses in a new way and ask themselves, *What part of this can I do?*

They couldn't do Warrior II, so I showed them how to use folding chairs so they could prop their thighs; then they could do it. They learned that they could use the wall to take some of their weight. I taught them how to be in their bodies—active feet, Ujjayi breathing—

even though I didn't even know how to be in my own body. They could do a whole lot more than any of us thought they could; we just had to get creative. As I worked to accommodate their limitations, the voice inside me droning *they're fat/they smell/you're gonna get it* began to quiet, and I began to get in touch with this struggling, suffering being I found inside each of them. We were the same! I gained so much respect for these women and their courage.

Learning to ask the question—*What part of this can I do?*—changed my life that day and every day I remember to ask it. Learning to work within the women's limitations gave me a powerful foundation for my future work with people who were injured, paralyzed, or in wheelchairs. I learned later from the director of the ranch that my Yoga students began participating in other activities as well; their confidence from the class had begun to spill into the rest of their lives. For me, this was the beginning of understanding that Yoga happens both on and off the mat.

My students helped me by allowing me to help them with their problems. I developed a tiny bit of self-respect because I was able to get over my fear of touching and moving them around and making them sweat. That was huge for me. I'd taught them that they could do something with their bodies besides haul them around, hate them, and shove food down them. Maybe I could learn the same for myself.

Every day my body became healthier as the toxins leached from it and I brought more Yoga healing into it. I could feel that I had a gift for Yoga—both learning and teaching the poses as well as metabolizing the wisdom of it.

Near the end of my stay, some locals pointed out magic mushrooms growing in the cow patties in the pastures near the ranch. Here was a natural high, just there for the picking. But I refused to touch them. I'd taken a pledge to stay away from drugs and pills and booze, and turning down mushrooms was a way of honoring myself. That's how much I'd grown.

When I left my teacher training at the end of that month, I was clean, sober, and free from cigarettes for the first time since I was six years old. And I knew I was a healer. I'd gone from wanting to die to having something to live for. For the first time ever, I was choosing life.

CHOOSING LIFE

It's not enough to die and be reborn; you must set your intent and choose life. Every day.

The Death Meditation may have given you the opportunity for a crucial reckoning. Perhaps the contemplation of death wasn't metaphorical; you've been there. A lot of students come to me so badly damaged that asking them to choose life is like asking them to flap their wings and fly to the moon. Can't be done.

When Frances, a be-ringed and heavily tattooed Yoga student, first came to me, she was struggling to overcome an abusive childhood. Sullen and shut down, she'd tried committing suicide any number of ways, including the slow methods of drugs, eating disorders, and cutting. The first time I put my hands on her to make an adjustment, she cringed and flinched; hands on her meant something really bad, even though the child in her yearned for a comforting touch. "Frances, you're safe here," I told her, and she began to cry, the beginning of a breakthrough.

But before the healing came storm after storm after storm. I taught her how to ride the waves, telling her, "Choose life. Frances, you've got to choose life." That became Frances's mantra. It was a long, slow road: she had to learn to trust me a little, then to trust herself a little, then to put some trust in living. She started taking massage training classes and apprenticed with me. I'd tell her, "Okay, you put your hands on this person along with me, match my energy." Then, slowly, slowly, she began to care about the people she was touching . . . and then herself. Underneath that tough, growly exterior, she discovered that she had the energy of a great healer. Today Frances has two viable careers—massage and Yoga.

WHAT DO YOU YEARN FOR?

What is your heart's desire? What do you yearn to do in the world? *Desire* and *yearn* are strong, important words that have such baggage around them. Desire was a slippery concept for me; it was a blank spot in my life, something I didn't notice that I didn't notice. If I even allowed myself to admit that there was something I yearned for, the voices would start up the chorus inside me: *That's impossible. You're wrong to want it. A cancerous scab like you could never do that. You can't ever have what you want.* Another problem is that desire is a big, bad no-no in traditional Yoga culture. The only desires you're allowed are PC ones, like enlightenment and world peace.

A lot of our culture's Judeo-Christian beliefs are conditioned against desire. We're taught that to make ourselves so-called better persons, we must behave altruistically, which in this case means always putting others first and negating our own desires. A lot of us are taught this so we better fit into the fabric of society. No wonder we have so much difficulty discerning our heart's desire; we have to cut through a lot of well-intentioned yet stupid teaching to find out what it is. But if we learn to follow our heart's desire and can get through the initial blowback, if we're taught to follow our Spirit's calling, how could that not be a tremendous gift to our family and community? Yes, sometimes following our heart's desire leads us into some crazy-ass places, but that's just part of it.

To discover what we truly desire, we must first strip away what we've been taught to desire: a certain weight, certain clothing, a certain mate, all those things that show that we're successful and happy. Out of love and concern, your parents might have inadvertently imposed their desires on you, encouraging you to become a doctor or to make a certain amount of money rather than to follow your innate gifts and skills.

We must return to the desires we've buried deep inside because we felt we didn't deserve them or couldn't have them. We have to look beyond surfaces and discern a true desire. Perhaps you think you want to be really rich, but what you really desire is to live free from fear of want. Maybe you think you want to screw all night, but what you really desire is a deep, ecstatic connection.

The beauty of the Death Meditation is that it strips everything away, leaving you with clarity about your deepest regrets—*I never got to write that book. I never became a teacher.* Your regrets can help you track and hunt your heart and Spirit's desire. My evolution has been in direct proportion to my ability to ask good questions: *What does it mean to be human? If I'm going to be on this planet, where is home?* Go on a quest to find your own purpose, your own home.

The Death Meditation allowed you to separate all those noble responsibilities—*I must pay the mortgage. I must raise my kids. I must care for my ailing parents.*—and focus instead on the dreams that got buried. We carry much more than we are actually responsible for. The sweetness of the Death Meditation is that it lets us look at the unnecessary weight on our shoulders and know we must lay it down in order to pursue our true desires. And it gives us the courage to do so.

Now it's time to take the next step.

SPIRITUAL FOCUS:
SET YOUR INTENT

The path you'll need to walk to achieve your goals is a long one. It's easy to lose focus. That's why it's so important to set your intent every day. Renew your commitment to live life authentically daily. Most of us wake up, toss some coffee down our throats, and rush headlong into our day. Instead, if you pause to begin your day with a strong intent about what you plan to discover or why you'll take a certain action, you'll get better results. You can go out in the wilderness and wander, or you can go out and start tracking.

This doesn't need to be an elaborate song and dance; I set my intent in the shower every morning. I stand in simple ceremony as the water pours over my head: I close my eyes and first picture cleansing white water rushing over me. Then I visualize the lavender hue the water takes on during certain stormy skies and picture that cascade cleansing my karma, the actions I take in this life. Finally, I visualize that gorgeous silver-gold-orange hue when the sun is setting on the water, and I imagine it washing over me. For me, that's the symbol of prosperity. I don't mean prosperity as in abundance of gold or money. I ask for the prosperity of good health, of being able to tap in to my creativity, of an abundance of students who can learn from me, of love and time enough for love. That's real richness.

By now I've woken up a little bit. Then I ask: *What would be meaningful for me to do today? How do I want to live this day?* Setting intent isn't simply making a list of things to do. It's asking yourself: *What action step do I need to take to walk into the person I most want to be? What's the quality of energy I want in my life today, no matter what I do? Exhil-*

aration? Quiet contemplation? I choose heightened awareness, so I go through the day with eyes wide open instead of on autopilot.

If you're looking for quiet contemplation, your intent might be to take a moment once every hour to absorb something in Beauty. Or to breathe steadily throughout the day. If instead you crave heightened awareness, can you set the intent of stopping every hour to do shoulder shrugs, so you put yourself back in your body? Or pet the cat for a few minutes every hour to feel that softness and connect to the loving energy of a four-feet? That Sweet Medicine (as Native Americans call the animal world) can have a profound effect on us, shifting us chemically, internally, spiritually. Setting your intent helps you break habits of mind that hold you back. We all tend to clench and tighten internally during scary moments; then we make a fear-based decision that we'll regret. Instead, can you set your intent to stop and breathe through that scary moment? If you're someone who gets easily flummoxed every time you hit an obstacle, can you set your intent not to have an expectation that says, *I have to solve this problem immediately in a brilliant way*? That way you allow yourself some flexibility to problem solve instead of going into despair and paralysis. Then simply place your hand on your heart and breathe in something that nourishes you with Beauty.

If you've got something in you that needs healing, your intent can be to breathe healing energy into that area, as many times a day as possible. If your priority is fitness, set your intent to take a walk around the block even though your brain says you can't afford the time.

Be flexible. Some people work better with bookend boundaries as action steps—*I will do this ten times*. Others prefer to repeat an action step however many times it feels comfortable in the moment. Pick whichever approach feels better to you. But give yourself a generous allowance. If your intention is to do Yoga every day, but you define doing Yoga as two hours of sweating during which you raise your heart rate for twenty minutes, then anything less than that can feel like a failure. When I injured my ankle, I couldn't meet my own definition of doing Yoga for a month and a half; I had to find other poses, use supports, do a lot of inversions.

Make your intent focused and doable. One of my students announced, "I want to be conscious and present 24-7." Even the Dalai

Lama would struggle with that one! I asked her to consider a different intent: "I want to be conscious for a whole breath." That was a sufficiently ambitious goal for her right them; she could stay conscious on the inhale but her mind flickered on the exhale. She'd get there with practice. If you're a parent who dreams of building a richer relationship with family, your intent might be to give each family member a quality moment, including yourself. Enjoy and relish the complexity and depth of that relationship for five minutes. Make it such a ridiculously brief amount of time that you can achieve it.

What's your good intent? If you can't think of one, start by focusing on your breath. Set your intent that once an hour, you'll take ten deep breaths. What a simple but profound step!

DHARMA JOUSTS

When you're choosing a new life for yourself, you're bound to smack into the habits and pitfalls of your old life. Make a game or dharma joust out of whatever you need to exercise. I define *dharma* as "what you do with what's been done to you." A dharma joust is a little bit of a battle, a parlay, a match. When I had that horrible realization of abuse in Dolphin pose, my decision to use that moment as an opportunity to heal was a dharma joust. If you're stuck in people-pleaser gear and someone asks you, "Hey, could you please write for our kids' school bulletin because you're such a good writer?" it's a great dharma joust to reply, "No, thanks. I'm busy." When you feel that old buzz of "I have to do ___," take a moment to engage with that. What does it take for you to say, "No, I'm not going to obey that today"? Find ways of jousting that are exciting.

It can be tremendously energizing to disobey the conditioning with which you were raised. Recognize when a pattern doesn't serve you anymore and put it in a context that's more exciting: *I'm going to find a great place to say no and say it with all my heart. Ally* with that disobedient rebellious energy to help you break old patterns.

CREATE A PRACTICE

Make change a practiced skill. Whatever it is you yearn to do or be, you must practice it, study it, or teach it—at least one of the three—every day. If you want to be a writer, you might not write every day, but you'll do something daily to further that intention, perhaps read a favorite author and investigate what it is about this writer that you love—that's research. That's part of the daily practice of working toward your dream or your goal.

Look at the notes from your Death Meditation every day to remind yourself of what you're choosing to weave, to make your actions part of what will build the masterpiece you want to make of your life. Create a practice that is doable no matter your health, age, weight, or energy level every day. What can you do *today* no matter what else is going on with you? What actions will you take to create the energy you'll need to accomplish that step?

How fun to think about what you'll need to become the person you most desire. If you want to get a horse, it's fun to think about where to start riding. If you dream of becoming a writer, it's fun to think about finding a writing buddy and setting up a weekly meeting to check in on each other's progress. If you long to become a Yoga teacher, it's fun to think about where to take teacher training. What is a step that brings you into that world?

For now, be six years old, making up a story without the adult parameters of perfectionism. Be playful versus professional. Your task now is to get the juices flowing; if you don't have foreplay, it ain't gonna happen. Do Lunge pose (see page 29) to open up your thighs and pelvis, or Handstand (see page 33). Hang your head upside down and give yourself a brain wash instead of being blocked. Move your body out of the chair.

This is where a to-do list helps. Writing down, *What must I do today to become this person I desire to be?* will keep you focused. Put your actions for your life practice at the top of your to-do list. Maybe your list will read: *Get up, brush teeth, write for twenty minutes.* Put your life practice right into your daily schedule.

The things that are most important to you might take seven weeks or maybe even seven years, but make sure you put action steps toward those longer-term goals on your daily to-do list. Consider the tasks before you. They're a bowl of beautiful stones—hematite, rose quartz, pyrite, lapis lazuli, jasper. Which one do you want to work on first? The most compelling one, or the easiest one as a warm-up to lubricate those synapses? Which do you have the propensity today to work on? They all need to be done, but in what sequence?

You've got seven million things to do; six aren't that important, but they're like loose wires whipping around. Sometimes creating order on this external level helps something settle inside of you. Choose a few from that loose-wire list and the time limit you'll spend on them. Maybe you'll devote an hour, maximum, to three things that have been bugging you on that list. That grubby light switch? It's not a big thing, but every time you notice it, it gives you a little *ping* of annoyance. Take five minutes and clean it so you get that hit of accomplishment. The next time you reach for that light switch to make a situation brighter, it won't be all grungy—that's a powerful metaphor.

Set up a winning process. If you do one thing on your list, that's a win. Acknowledge the win. Howl at the moon. Let's redefine what a win is. A win is an actual accomplishment, no matter the size. If your dream is to write a book, open up a file on your computer and call it *My Book*. You just created a doorway; that's a win.

If you're in a very dark place and taking even the smallest step seems like too much, be easy on yourself. Start really simply. If you're depressed, doing almost anything can be overwhelming. Can you take some deep breaths, and then get up and brush your hair? That might be it; that's a win. Can you get up and hang in a standing forward bend, breathing deeply, to bathe your brain in fresh blood and oxygen so you feel less lethargic? Can you feed yourself a meal that's good for you instead of simply filling the gaping hole in your belly? All wins. Be willing to honor those daily living steps as well as the bigger overview of connecting to your Spirit. Maybe all you can do is put your hand on your heart and take one deep breath. That's a damn good practice for the day. That super-simple act is a huge win.

BUILD A TRIBE THAT SUPPORTS YOU

Once you're on your new path, surround yourself with people who share a similar interest. If you want to be a writer, go to a writing class or convention. If you want to be an animal trainer, find one and ask if you can shadow her to see how it's done. Hang out with people who love the energy of change.

Separate yourself from fearful people. I'd been growing my career as a Yoga teacher for several years when I went back to visit my blood family. My brother and mother immediately started challenging me: "How could you charge so much for a single class?" I was with them for only a few hours, but they were already pushing my buttons. My income dropped for six months after that!

Don't hang out with people who lack a curiosity about life's path. Dealing with your own stuff is plenty hard enough, much less other people's. Do these people feed your fire for developing your heart's desire, or diminish it? Do they feed your belief that you can do it, or not? If not, cut off or change the relationship—quick!—before they infect you with their soul-deadening virus.

Right after I left the Yoga teacher training in Guadalajara, clean and sober, I went to visit my horse buddies. For these hard-partying druggies, the new me who didn't drink or smoke or do drugs was suspicious and uncomfortable to be around. I got a constant barrage of "Oh, here, have some vodka . . . oh, that's right; you don't drink anymore." They didn't like my new behavior because it challenged their decision not to change. We were no longer on common ground. I personally wasn't strong enough to sustain those relationships and stay sober, so in order to heal, I had to cut them off. In making that healing choice, I realized I was stronger than I'd thought.

The minutes of your life are precious. You want your time to be richly spent. Don't allow your life force to be drained by people who want to keep you in old patterns because the new ones make them uncomfortable. When you change, you're holding up a mirror to their lives too. If you're not drinking, it throws their drinking into a scary, glaring spotlight.

Change can be really sexy and exciting. If you're with other quantum leapers, every time they see you take a leap, they'll do a celebration dance. They won't say, "You only jumped six feet instead of twelve, you loser." You need people who can reflect your wins. But more importantly, you have to recognize the wins yourself. That expands your exploration of what's possible.

The environment you set up around your newly evolving self is crucial. Protect the newly growing bud of yourself. You wouldn't grow an orchid and then set that delicate, rare flower outside in a hailstorm. You are that: tender, unique, worth caring for through the cycle of creation, fallowness, flowering. Nurture yourself daily.

PHYSICAL FOCUS:
MEDITATION

The Death Meditation asked you to clarify what matters to you, what you want to focus on as you move forward. Setting your intent daily helps guide you on the path to that treasure. If you want to bring an even greater quality of attention to your day, meditation is an invaluable tool. A simple meditation practice is as cleansing and necessary as brushing one's teeth—and it need not be any more complicated.

Meditation is simply a way to shift the gears of the mind. We think a *lot.* And we think that's the only gear that the brain has, but it's more like first gear in a six-gear car. Many people think the goal of meditation is to shut down the mind. Not so; that just sets you up for war. Meditation is about exploring and teaching your mind to do something different; that's much more friendly than saying, *I'm gonna shut you up!* It's not about putting yourself to sleep; it's about awakening, especially awakening parts of you that have never been asked to awaken before. That's exciting and intriguing.

STARTING SIMPLE: TRACKING THROUGH FEELING

When I first started meditating, all the traditional rules flummoxed me—*Sit still! Focus on that mantra! Don't change your posture!* When I first tried to be still, my muscles would start to twitch and itch and spasm. Then I'd get into a different kind of war—*Oh, my back hurts!* I'd want to move, but the rules said, *Don't move.* It's easy to get tangled up in all those rules. I was studying martial arts once, and the instructor taught us some maneuver. "What do we use that move for?" I asked. He didn't know. I went on a hunt and found the answer in some moldy old book; the move was for monks to kick their long robes out of the way. That might have flown for monks in ancient times, but it's irrelevant now. If you want to make meditation a regular practice, you've got to find a way that makes sense for you. That may mean drop-kicking some of the rules.

Some folks have found that repeating a mantra—a very specific phrase—helps them because it gives the mind something to chatter about, so it occupies the part that thinks it needs to think. That form of meditation never worked for me; *om mani padme hum* became *ohwhatthefuckfor*. I have no problem with it; I just work a different way. But if your mind just can't shut up because it's so used to thought output, by all means, try a mantra. Simply focus on a word or phrase—*love* or *one*—as you breathe in and out.

What worked for me was to feel my breath. Listening for and feeling the music of my breath was very compelling when I let myself get interested in it, and it eventually made me brighter and brighter.

I began to meditate through motion, Yoga poses, doing something that sent the blood coursing through me. I started entertaining the concept of using my breath to track through feeling. I'd settle into a Yoga pose, say, Warrior I, then push through my foot, and ask myself, *Can I feel that?* Maybe I could feel my foot muscles, but not the calf or thigh. I'd go hunting for that physiological feeling next. This kind of meditation was teaching my mind to be alert, quiet, and perceptive. Slowly I was able to move into sitting meditations. Try this approach if sitting still is too difficult.

When you're starting out, choose an amount of time to stay quiet that's easy to accept. Maybe it's five minutes at first. That's a decent sit time. If everyone practiced sitting still and breathing for five minutes, that would be a helpful pause for business. For most people, to sit for twenty minutes is a long time. If all you can do is fret about how uncomfortable you are, you probably won't come back to it. It's more important to establish a daily practice where you can rest and be nourished. That's your Spirit's cup of coffee every day.

Find a place away from the usual distractions: phone, computer, loved ones. Put up a Do Not Disturb sign if you have to. This is your time.

If you're doing a sitting meditation, choose a firm chair (preferably one where you don't lean on the back for support, which can collapse and dull the spine) or place a cushion on the floor and sit so that you can keep your spine straight, your collarbones lifted, your shoulder blades relaxing down the back ribs, and the back of your skull lined up over the sacrum. This posture allows your chest to expand easily, which allows the freest passage of energy through the body.

Close your eyes and begin deep Ujjayi breathing. Let the mind rest but not sleep. Make the breath gentle, as effortless as possible, deep and steady with that soothing Ujjayi sound. Focus on feeling your deep breathing. Feel your ribs expanding, how your belly moves with your breath, how the air moves in and out of your nose (breathe through your mouth if you need to).

Meditation is like sitting on a bench watching cars go by. If a red car goes by, you don't have to jump up and chase it. Thoughts will come up, but you don't have to chase them. Keep a pad and paper next to you, so that if all those little to-dos come up, you can simply jot them down— *Call Betsy at 10:00 A.M.*—instead of going to war with your brain's honorable attempt to do its job of being responsible. Thank your brain for doing its job, write the damn thing down so you don't have to waste the time and energy dealing with it, and return to your breathing.

Get curious about the sensations you feel while breathing. Feel how the mind relaxes. Shift from *thinkthinkthink* to *ah, that's a nice feeling.* Not a shutdown, but an awake place. What do you feel when you have no input? You're just hanging out with whoever and whatever you are. That person is very mysterious; you don't know much about that person, which can be a fun thing. Instead of thinking, *I'm supposed to have these great insights but all I have is a numb butt,* tell yourself, *Cool! I'm gonna spend five minutes hanging out with the mystery of myself.*

Instead of looking for what is supposed to happen, put the supposes aside. What does it feel like to sit quietly and be with yourself, whatever that means, for a few minutes? Let the deep breathing in your meditation nourish and recharge you. This isn't a place to work much of anything out. It's a time to simply drink in the sweetness and essence of the cosmos, feeling for the truth that you are a part of it, no matter what your self-mutilating thoughts and beliefs are. When you sit for the first five hundred times, maybe all you can drink in is your breath. That's spectacular! There's not a good meditation and a bad meditation—it's all good grist for the mill. If you sit, that's a win. Sometimes you'll have moments of sweet quiet; other times you'll be in list-making mode. We judge ourselves really harshly. Put that aside; it's not helpful.

Sometimes I'll do what I call doctoring while I'm sitting. If your back starts to hurt, you can breathe into that place. Be curious and fascinated. Ask, *What does that do?* Or break another rule: don't sit there and suffer; allow yourself sixty seconds to do something about it—hang over in forward bend or Neck Release (see page 64) poses. I think that's an absolutely acceptable meditation. If your brain is all jumpy and agitated and then suddenly narcoleptic, breathe into your brain. That's easy—your nose is hooked right up to the brain. Feed the brain oxygen, not thoughts. Don't get so rigid: *Oh, if I think about feeding my brain, that's a thought.* Yes it is. Take the action anyway. You won't be free of thought, but you're teaching your mind to be at rest. If you have emotional heartbreak, just breathe into that area, being willing to let whatever layers or tightness are there unfold. Feel what happens. It's like watching waves crest on the ocean: build, crest, break, withdraw, repeat. We all carry extra weight in our hearts; we can all stand to unload and oxygenate more. That's a sweet overall practice.

I find it helpful to know when my sitting is beginning and ending. Some people bow in namaste at the end of their practice, a way of saying, *Thank you for the practice.* I'll bring my hands together and charge them—feel that molecular bonding of energy warming them—and then put them on my knees for a while. I'll close by saying, "Thank you," or, "Aho. *Mitakuye Oyasin,*" which is Lakota for "All my relations" or "In celebration of all the people." I like to tap my drum three times at the beginning and three times at the end of a meditation. Some people like bells. Sometimes I do simple Native American chants, like the Cherokee Morning Song. Experiment with what works for you. Take a few moments, feel the benefits, subtle and obvious.

BRAHMARI—GET BUZZED UP FOR MEDITATION BY ALIGNING YOUR CHAKRAS

If you want to add an exciting layer onto your meditation, I recommend Brahmari breathing, sometimes called bee breath because it makes a buzzing sound. I like to do a round of Brahmari breathing through all my chakras before I begin my meditation because it gets all these different parts of me turned on and alive, and I want my body fully alert to support my brain.

Chakras are very simply the energy and information centers that run through the body from crotch to crown. Some people talk about 144 chakras; I'm talking about the basic seven from the top of the head to the bottom of the pelvis. Brahmari breathing is a simple focusing exercise that will help you activate and align each of these seven centers.

Begin by inhaling deeply through the nose. With your exhale, buzz with your lips softly closed. You'll sound like a very large, buzzing bee. Play with the buzz; the higher the pitch, the more it moves up in the body. The lower the pitch, the easier it is to move it down. When I need to buzz up my brain because it feels smoggy or sluggish or disconnected, I'll do some high-pitched buzzes to get into the seventh and sixth chakras, but it's really best to go through all seven chakras. Aim for a minimum of three breaths into each chakra. It takes me at least two breaths to get me where I'm going with my Brahmari. Relax while you do this; there's no particular timeline.

Start at the seventh or Crown chakra at the top of the head. We start at the top and go down because it's easier to buzz into your head with your nose right there. This area, right on top of your brain and pituitary gland, is a place of overview. Ask, *What is my purpose or mission here in this lifetime?* The seventh chakra is where you begin to connect with your unique gifts to offer the world as well as the gifts you want to develop for yourself. Put your fingertips or hands on top of your head so you can feel whether your skull is vibrating, as if you've plucked a harp string. With each exhale, which should be as long and drawn out as possible, do a high-pitched buzzing until you're completely out of breath. With each inhale, feel for washing the breath right from the nostrils into the brain, sending a cleansing wind over the brain, blowing out the cobwebs, sleepiness, fogginess. Do that for three breaths.

Now put your arms down, take a breath into the sixth chakra, which includes the eyes and ears, ocular muscles and inner ears, bottom and back of the brain, and the pineal gland. This is the place of insight— where you literally see inward and hear your intuition, the voice of your Spirit. This is the place where you start to tap in to your inner guidance, the wisdom that tells you what to do. I once heard this internal voice say, *Turn right at the next corner,* while I was driving. I ignored it, even though it was really clear. I kept plowing straight ahead and promptly ran into a roadblock with police at some weird checkpoint. Chances are if I'd turned right, I would have avoided it. How often do we ignore those inner promptings? Let's start listening to them instead.

Take your two middle fingers and lay them gently on your eyeballs, with your thumbs over your earflaps to plug your ears. This helps you focus more deeply inside your brain. Sometimes you'll even see a blurry blob that brightens as you do your buzzing breath. Slightly, slightly lower the pitch of your buzzing. Use your breath to play with the pitch; is it buzzing close to the area you want? Take three Brahmari breaths.

Then move to the fifth chakra, which governs your neck, throat, thyroid, jaw, and mouth—one of the places for Truth Speaking, for voicing your opinions, your emotions. Ask internally, *What's truly important, what matters to me the most?* How does your throat area feel? Are you choking it back because it's been devalued? Do you have temporomandibular joint disorder (TMJ)? If so, you'll want to put special attention to this area. Put your hands on your throat or lightly on the sides of the jaw or maybe a hand on the back of the neck. Relax the jaw; move your lower teeth off the upper teeth. Begin your Brahmari breathing. Your lips may vibrate and tickle, or you may feel a funny, buzzy sensation in the jaw, or your chin may tremble—that's good tracking. If the Brahmari irritates the throat, go gentle; take a swallow of water. Give it three buzzy breaths.

Now for the fourth chakra, connected to the heart, lungs, bronchial tubes, lymph glands in the armpits, shoulders, and the whole upper back. The back of the heart area ranges from the bottom tips of the shoulder blades to the base of the neck, from the mid-ribcage up to collarbone and your thymus, which informs the Warrior's Heart. It's part of the immune system. The fourth chakra is a place of love, compassionate wisdom, how we care for and about ourselves and others. It's a place of heart truth and discernment, which is why it has to be aligned with the brain—the discernment of the brain must work with the compassionate wisdom of the heart.

To access this area, cross your arms and put your right hand in your left armpit and your left hand in your right armpit. Others prefer to put their hands over their breast bone or heart. Find out what helps you connect. Slightly lower your pitch by relaxing your voice so it deepens a little. It should feel like you're opening the chambers of the heart when you get really good at it, but just feeling your ribs open as you buzz-breathe is great. Keep it simple. Feel the buzz. Take three luxurious breaths.

The third chakra connects to the belly, diaphragm, lower ribs, liver, spleen, gall bladder, pancreas, kidneys, and adrenal glands. The stomach is where information collects; when something attacks you emotionally, you feel it like a blow in the belly. To access this area, put your hands on your solar plexus or on your sides at the bottom ribs so you can really feel a deeper, expanding breath. If you have pain in the lower back, put your hand there; this is the time to buzz it up. Relax your breath so you can get a deeper buzz, and give it three deep, long breaths.

The second chakra connects to the intestines, top of the pelvis, lower back and sacrum, uterus, ovaries, fallopian tubes, prostate gland, and bladder. In Native American Medicine, the uterus, a place of women's magic, is the Great Mystery because creation happens there. Creation and ensoulment are mysterious. At the same time, the intestines are where the body discerns what is nutritive and what needs to be passed on as waste.

We have the same problem in our culture as we do in our bodies: we take in too much that's nonnutritive, whether it's junk food or junk information, and we attempt to be fed by it. We pour in so much information, so much food, and our bodies and minds and emotions get constipated, clogged, overloaded. What the hell is in an energy drink, and what is our cell tissue going to do with it? Of the information we take in, how much of it can we actually live on and how much is crap? There's nothing wrong with crap, but it's an end product. Literally: eat shit and die.

The alternative: buzz up the area, turn it on, and learn discernment. Then balloon your breath down. On the inhale, feel the diaphragm spreading and pressing down. Feel the low belly moving down—the top rim of the sacrum moves away from the spinal cord as you acquire skill for this. Take three deeply pitched buzzing breaths.

Now for the first chakra. Have you ever noticed that when you get really scared, you numb out in your pelvis or your sphincter tightens? Fear and security have to do with this area, including the bottom of the colon and the pelvic bowl, which are the roots of sexuality and life force—where the fires of your immune system are. If your fires are dim in this area, so is your immune system. If you spend your life in a chair, it weakens your immune system.

What we're taught about being a woman or a man or sexual or desirable—all of that can shut our pelvis down. When society tells women, "Don't feel your vagina!" it's crippling. We are dampening our creativity, our life force, our core strength—that's deadly! We lose so much by obeying those teachings. For those of us who have had trauma, that shuts the area down as well, with heavy repercussions for the rest of our bodies—our immune system, creativity, love, faith. Some people who may be numb in that area are able to start a secondary fire in their heart, but without that basic magma core, they miss some of the grounding energy necessary to physically manifest their creation. If you can restore that core fire, that magma, that heartbeat of the earth, what would be ignited in your creativity, your cell structure, your body's ability to cleanse and renew itself? This is a very primal place: life, sex, security, procreation, species survival, shelter. It's where the flames of the life force are.

Buzzing into the first chakra can be scary since you're tapping into that power, sexuality, life-and-death stuff—if you've got no food, no shelter, you're dead meat. Can you have a blast with coming alive instead? As you inhale, balloon your breath down into the anus and perineum, pressing the genitals against the chair. Feel how odd that feels—whoo! (Similar to women, sometimes men, in an attempt to be good by society's standards, cut off the energy to their genitals. They castrate themselves. Men, be reassured: we love your sexuality. Just learn to use it appropriately.)

If you were playing the chakras like a guitar, the first chakra would be your low E string. Where is your resonance? Feel for it. If I make a really loud Brahmari, I miss it. If I go into the deep yet subtle, sometimes I can sink into atomic awareness, seeing and feeling the proton-neutron dance—the tremendous amount of movement that goes on at the cellular level. I see that I'm made out of a cosmos of space with these tiny little particles moving in an intelligent dance to form a certain pattern.

Recognizing that truth—that this is how we are made—the response changes from *I don't want to feel my vagina/anus* to *Who is designing the dance? Who did the choreography? Can I learn to be my own choreographer?* What amazing Beauty, to see that brilliant dance, to take my awareness down to that level—to feel and ask, *What is my first chakra's resonance?* These questions are a lot more fun to play with. When you buzz, you have to feel for that ever-so-subtle response. The area isn't used to responding, so it may be a little sleepy. Even the slightest feeling means you're on the right track.

When you buzz the first chakra, it helps to keep a little downward pressure using the abdominals. Not hard, not struggling—just lean a little into the area in a friendly way. I think of it as snuggling up to it. I know it's appalling to many to think of snuggling up to your own anus and genitals—but when we get friendly with that area, it makes a huge difference in our lives almost immediately. We need that friendliness toward ourselves.

Next time you go to your computer, sit down and take a few breaths into your first chakra, activating that creativity. Not only will it keep your ass from going numb, but it will fill you with aliveness.

The length of buzzing through the chakras will vary depending on your inhalation and exhalation. The first time might take you twenty minutes. Luxuriate in the length of your inhale and exhale. Don't do the New York–Minute approach—*Oh, I'll just take one breath into each area*—you're setting yourself up for a failure. It takes three breaths minimum to get into each area. If you get even an inkling of turning on the energy there, that's your great beginning. You've established your connection through feeling and made a doorway.

AFTER YOU SIT

Ideally, you'll start your day by setting your intent, turning on your chakras with your Brahmari breathing, and meditating for a few minutes.

After your meditation, take another thirty seconds or minute to sit again with your intent. Can you get any more specific with it? The more specific it is, the more doable it is. *I want to be kind today* might become *I will put aside my judgments of* _____. Can you include yourself in that kindness? If you're in a challenging situation with another person, ask,

What is the kindest true thing I can do or say right now for myself or this other? The only answer might be: *Take a breath. Put your hand on your heart. Or theirs.* Start with small, doable steps and experiment with how they feel to you.

Check your energy level and decide: where are you going to be most effective and efficient today? If you force it without first making that connection, the work will be missing its soul. Stay alert to all the sneaky ways you can indulge in your avoidances. Perhaps you promised yourself that you'd go to the gym after work, but you're just getting over a cold and you've got an insanely busy day ahead. Can you reset your intent and commit to going to the gym for at least a half hour and doing some part of your routine and then reassessing how that feels? Or maybe there's a scary thing you're putting off. Can you commit to reassessing that situation after a half hour? Maybe you can do some of it.

Medicine People teach that after ceremony, you walk with a different wide-open perception, but after a while, you fade into your normal mode of perception. After meditation, check and reset your intent. How can you incorporate any realizations or breakthroughs you've had and make them meaningful in your life today? For example, my meditation, commitment, and intent was to bring my health into balance, specifically my endocrine system. Regular blood tests gave me hard evidence to assess whether whatever I was doing was working and how to self-correct. This invaluable information helped me reset my intent. Having tangible steps gives so much more power, richness, purpose, and success to your life.

Who do you yearn to become? How does that person move, talk, breathe, feel, and make love? Picture that beautiful, intuitively wise person. How will you build the road from where you are now to where that person is standing? Embodying a human takes a lot of practice, experimentation, and failure, but that's the only way to get to that person you most yearn to become. Set your intent. Practice, experiment, fail, do something different. Meditate to bring your attention to what lights you up. Both your successes and failures will help you discover something new, which is what will take you forward.

6

HUNGER PAINS:
LEARNING TO LISTEN WITHIN

I LOOKED AT the clock: nine P.M. Finally, it was time. I was home alone, so no one would see me; I wouldn't have to cower in the tiny bedroom off the bathroom or in the storage room. I'd been planning this moment, thinking about what I was going to do a hundred times throughout the day. I was ready.

I started in on the leftover tofu lasagna. There was three-quarters of the pan left, made of the finest organic products. I shoveled it all in with my bare hands, too eager and starving to bother with reheating it. Then macrobiotic rice and beans still warm from the Crock-Pot. It was nasty looking, like a cow afterbirth, but I made short work of it. Then a few strawberries, some chunks of pineapple, an apple. Once I started to eat, I'd become more and more indiscriminate. What else was in the fridge? A block of tofu. A second and third block. I wolfed them down while crouching on the floor in front of the open fridge. Then some cooked vegetables. Then some ice cream and cheesecake. The more I ate, the deeper into trance I went. Numb, like when I'd gotten drunk as a toddler on the floor near the liquor cabinet. My stomach hurt, but only from a dull distance, as if it didn't even belong to me. I didn't really feel anything, except the tightness of the skin over my belly.

I walked down the hall and knelt in front of the toilet. At first I'd needed the finger down my throat, but now I could just concentrate and do a reverse swallow. I couldn't help but see the humor in my situation. I'd spent so much time painstakingly preparing all this expensive organic food, soaking all the beans and almonds. It took hours and hours to prepare, but just minutes to eat it and puke it out.

I liked the more immediate methodology; laxatives were just too slow. As the toilet bowl filled, I told myself I was just a goat chewing my cud, bringing it up in reverse. I was dimly aware of a steady undercurrent of disgust, but the puking felt like a purge of even that. *Gotta get it out. Get it out. Get it out.* There. Relief. The effort was exhausting, which was useful. I curled up in front of the wall heater for a few hours, then lay down on the couch to read for a bit, then did a little Yoga. Then back to the kitchen to start the cycle all over again. Finally, at about three or four in the morning, I was tired enough to fall asleep.

The next morning I woke up exhausted, my throat sore. I could barely lift my head. When I looked in the mirror, these dead red eyes stared back at me; I'd burst all the blood vessels in them by puking. It wasn't until I took a drink of water and it bounced right back up and out, as if it had hit a trampoline, that I began to think maybe I had a little problem.

Two years earlier, making my decision to choose life and get my Yoga teaching certification had been a gigantic step toward healing, but I was still a very broken person. I didn't have any idea what to do after I'd finished my training. I didn't even have any money to leave Mexico! Some of the people in the course pooled their money to buy me a ticket back to L.A. Once we arrived, these two women I was traveling with said, "Well, where're you going?"

"I don't know. Just drop me off at the Center for Yoga." I'd taken classes there, and I knew some of the folks who worked there. I walked in and, putting on my best fake confident facade, said, "Hi, I just finished the teacher training and I thought you could use some help here." The staff let me teach, clean, whatever I could do. By the time the owners—Ganga and his wife, Lily—came back from teaching and traveling, I was pretty firmly entrenched.

Day by day, I was still trying to find a reason to live and a way out of the hideous places inside my mind. As I kept practicing and teaching Yoga and my body started to loosen, I began to get a sense of freedom and power that I hadn't had before. That was wonderful, but it wasn't enough. I was hungry, but I didn't even know what I was craving.

I had read everything I could find about enlightenment. But the more I read, the more despair I went into because these texts had nothing to do with me and my problems. Enlightenment? I just wanted to wake up without wanting to kill myself. Each day was a battle to choose life.

All the Yoga philosophy was about transcending the body, which I interpreted as a damaging message: *We'll get rewarded after we die, so it doesn't matter how we wreck our planet or each other or our bodies.* I wanted to know: how do you live spiritually in your body on this earth? I was less interested in transcending this bag of hair, blood, shit, and bones.

My puking was a reflection of my state of mind. It'd gone into hiding while I was down in Mexico because there was miraculously an abundance of food every day. I'd gone from a panicky feeling that I'd starve to the trust that there would be breakfast, dinner, food always available. Even so, I was haunted by a sense that I didn't deserve it. One day I'd been on my way to the dining hall when a skunk barred my path and chased me away—more confirmation that I didn't deserve to eat. Now, while I worked at the Center for Yoga, eating and puking was steadily becoming the central feature of my days. I'd broken my addiction to alcohol, drugs, and cigarettes, but I'd really just traded my dependence on those addictions for another, more insidious one. From my earliest days, I'd always vomited—not surprising, given all the alcohol, drugs, and trauma I was ingesting. And I'd never had a good relationship with food: living with morbidly obese people can mess with your mind, especially when there's a padlock on the fridge (I never knew who put it there, or whether it was supposed to keep me or the rest of the family away) and your own family is stealing your food.

I could tell you down to the ounce how much to feed a horse when it's competing compared to when it's resting, but I had no clue how to feed myself. As a teenager, the puking had become more ritualized—it was one of the few bonding experiences I recalled sharing with my sister, a dancer who struggled to keep her weight down. You know you've got a twisted relationship when your warmest childhood memory is listening to your sister puke in the next stall in a restaurant restroom and realizing, "Hey, you do that too!"

I realized that bulimia was my body's attempt to fill a spiritual void and decided I needed to find other authorities who could show me the way. My relationship with Ganga, a wiry, compact man with a wild mane of curly brown hair and a trim mustache, became sexual after he and his wife split. Together we began to explore our spirituality. He convinced me that it would be a hip, fun thing for me to take a vow of poverty. We developed a system of double Yoga, in which all the poses are partnered, published a book, *Double Yoga,* and even did a small book tour. Ganga suggested we travel to India—the seat of enlightenment—to further our Yoga practice. Maybe chasing enlightenment would be as useless as the time Squirrel and I had raced to the end of the rainbow, but I went for it.

I was completely unprepared for the sheer press of humanity, the ever-present poverty, the stench, and rampant disease I found in India. In the mornings we'd sit for hour upon hour of lectures on homeopathy and naturopathy, and then in the afternoon the open clinic would throw wide its doors to anybody in India who had a problem. Some really nasty stuff crawled through those doors. Lepers, people with scabies, one guy who'd been attacked by wild dogs and whose wounds leaked pus. It was hardcore, but none of it seemed to faze our teacher, a very tiny, very round, very white, silver-haired Irish grandmother named Naryiani. She was all of 4'8" at most, yet this homeopathic healer poured her all into setting up clinics, training people, and treating anyone who needed her—all at no charge. I was blown away by that. Here we were surrounded by all these allegedly evolved people walking around in orange robes, trying to be holier than thou, and this little old lady just whipped their asses.

Sometimes Naryiani took me on some of her personal rounds. One day we went to see a dying swami, surrounded by all his acolytes. He sat on a kind of throne, looking gray and terribly ill. As he and my teacher conversed in English, he suddenly leaned closer to her and said, "Naryiani, I'm afraid to die." His acolytes freaked; he was supposed to be an enlightened master with an unshakable belief that death was merely a transition, yet here he was, confessing his fear to this white woman. And Naryiani just made a clucking noise, wrapped her arms around him, and brought his head into her breast, like a comforting mother. Now the acolytes *really* freaked out. A *woman* was touching their master, cradling him on her *breast,* and she was *white!* I was so impressed with her courage; she saw that this man desperately needed comfort, so she walked right past the rules of that spiritual order and gave his untouchable holiness the touch that he needed. She operated on pure intuition and love. No matter what the doctrine decreed, she would not let him be so alone in his death.

As I watched Naryiani bathe the most grievously ill people in her great Irish grandmaternal spirit, I learned the limits of where I wanted to direct my own powers of healing. It wasn't in me to minister to the lepers of the world; I didn't have that kind of courage. But from this small person with a huge heart, I learned a powerful lesson: you don't demonstrate your values by wrapping yourself in saffron cloth; you do it by your actions in daily living.

I loved studying and hanging out with the sadhus, the wild yogis of India. Through years of spiritual practice, these holy ones shed layer upon layer of attachments until they are literally stripped of everything but spirit and cow dung powder, living in caves or wandering from town to town with their long dreadlocks flying, their dark, wild, naked bodies covered head to toe with white ash. They're very strong people; they walk a lot. I sensed in them kindred spirits; like me, they'd chosen to exist on the edge of society. In fact, to the people of India, they were considered "dead unto themselves," and legally dead to the state. I empathized with living partway between the worlds of the living and the dead.

Next I sought out B. K. S. Iyengar, a legendary Yoga teacher. Millions had benefited from his wisdom, and I'd read his bestseller, *Light on Yoga,* so I was excited to go to his world-famous Yoga Institute in Pune, India, to study with the master. I'd been impressed by his emphasis on extreme precision in the poses; I knew that Iyengar teachers required special training, and I wanted to become one of them. What I didn't realize was that Iyengar accomplished his "active correction" through hitting, spitting, and screaming.

I put up with his truly bad behavior because, after all, he'd been teaching for more than forty years by then. He *had* to have all the answers I craved. Trials by fire didn't bother me; how many had I already lived through? I figured if I just put up with it, I'd pass the test and he'd give me the key. Iyengar did a lot of things to break me, such as pushing his toes hard into my diaphragm, but physical pain isn't how to break me; kindness is. He'd mock me constantly, calling me expert. "So, expert, finally you cry." "I have a cold, Mr. Iyengar," I sparred back. I'd had fifteen hundred pounds of horseflesh try to kill me; what could one small man really do? We both behaved childishly; he huffing and puffing, me willfully resisting. Whatever wisdom he had, he wasn't willing to give it to me because I hadn't agreed to his demand for subservience. At the end of the month-long training, we all lined up during the celebratory dinner to kneel before Iyengar and touch his feet. As I approached, he said, "Oh, so, expert, you have no need ever to come back here." And I replied, "Oh, I know that, Mr. Iyengar." I'd learned what I most needed to know: that I couldn't look to others for the wisdom that lay inside me.

Another breakthrough came when I was wandering in the mountains, walking along a path in the bright, hot sunlight, when I came upon a cave and entered it. As my eyes adjusted to the dimness, I realized it was full of people. There was a woman sadhu, dreadlocked and ash-covered royalty, with luminous liquid brown eyes. She sat on a smooth rock covered with some kind of skin, surrounded by men—an unusual situation in India, where women were treated as second-class citizens. She was obviously a woman of power, even in this land. I spoke to her in English, and she spoke in a language I couldn't understand. We talked for a long time—I, a daughter of Kali, she, one of the radiant ones. Something shifted inside me; I realized it was possible for me to be both wild and holy.

My travels through India were a crazy mix of mysticism and misery. Its rivers and mountains were home to me—in a literal sense I didn't quite understand but knew for sure. In India, magic was a daily reality spiced with the scent of the burning of dead bodies in the omnipresent ceremonial ghats. I was honored to be a student of Gangotri, one of the country's most brilliant and authentic magic sadhus. I felt the sadhus were my people, but the hordes of people, the teeming masses crawling with disease, freaked me out. One second I'd be smiling at a Brahma bull walking freely down the street, its milk-white hide painted in bright colors; the next moment someone would squat right next to me and take a crap. The filth and ignorance and illness were all too much for me. One day Ganga and I were eating in the Taj Mahal Palace hotel in Bombay— an incredibly garish five-star hotel, very expensive by Indian standards. We were sitting at the rich, elaborate buffet, eating our fill. I looked out the window and saw a woman dying in the gutter while I was gorging— that became my metaphor for India. What do you do with all the woes of the world?

When I returned to L.A. after my long travels, I came to see this period of my life as my traditional Yoga phase. I'd learned a great deal about being a healer, of course, and deepened my study of Iyengar Yoga before putting it aside. The holy healers I most admired were the ones who tossed out the rulebook and did their work from a deep, intuitive place—Naryiani, the sadhus, the magic wild woman. Whenever I tried to play by the rules—*You must do this posture exactly this way, or I'll hit you* or *If you want to be Enlightened, you must do xyz*—it fit badly, like stolen shoes. Something in me rebelled or sabotaged the situation. Whenever I listened to my intuition, I seemed able to take from my wisdom in life experience.

I'd continued my bingeing and purging throughout my travels in India, with no less control over it now that I was back in the United States. For years I'd been getting devoured alive during Dream-Time and had survived alcoholic blackouts so bad I'd wake up in strange places next to total strangers. I'd have to find a newspaper to find out what day and city I was in. So what was so weird about a little puking? I was proud of learning to throw up without using my fingers. It wasn't until Ganga gave me a tiny article that mentioned using enemas to purge that I learned a new word: bulimia. To this day, I don't know whether or not it was his way of letting me know that he was on to me and trying to help me, but I quickly decided that the word didn't apply to me. Enemas? Ew. Who would do that? Now *that* was screwed up.

The combination of my travels and my insights about authority began to shift something inside me. After my years of sobriety, Ganga and I experimented with doing pot, hash, mushrooms, and acid during *pranayama,* or breath work, to get into some new places. We were trying to follow the tradition of using these as sacred teacher plants, but it felt radically wrong. I'd read Carlos Castaneda and about other mystical traditions, but ending my sobriety was still scary for me. When I went to the dentist, I wouldn't even let him use Novocain when he was drilling into my jaw because I was so afraid it would throw me back into the drug world. But I wanted to see if this could bring me closer to enlightenment. But this wasn't the way for me. This wasn't the way to anything I wanted. I realized I had to learn to access those places without drugs.

Gradually I began to realize that as much as I had learned through our work and travels together, I was also suffocating under Ganga's influence. He collected all the money I'd made teaching Yoga. I received none of the proceeds from the book we'd done together; Ganga told me we were using it to pay for our trip to India. I even gave him the initial payment I got from a bit part in a movie called *Blue Thunder.* I was seriously rethinking this vow of poverty I'd taken.

I finally got to the point that I'd decided I'd rather shoot myself in the head than throw up one more time. I was sick of throwing so many hours of every day over to craving fantasies, trance eating, puking—I couldn't ever relax unless I'd gone through the entire ritual of bingeing and purging. I was sick of the tremendous physical effort—like running a marathon every day of my life. Here I was, teaching Yoga and life balance, and I was whacked from "talking to the dinosaurs on the big white porcelain phone" as bulimics like to joke.

My adventures in this traditional Yoga phase triggered an amazing epiphany about the connection between my puking and Ganga. My body was literally telling me, *I cannot stomach this relationship anymore.* It was time to listen to my own body, my own truths, and my own wisdom.

I had to go inside and find out what to do with what was going on.

HEALING MY BULIMIA

Learning to deal with my bulimia meant learning to listen to my body's real hunger. Each of us is hungry for something, but we'll never quell those hunger pains until we learn to stop blindly following the authorities outside ourselves, disobey the voices of our addiction, and instead start tuning in to something more compelling.

My process was trial and error. Eating disorders are the one addiction I couldn't simply cut out of my life. With my other substance abuse, I could use my very strong will to refuse to pick up the bottle or the tobacco. With bulimia, I couldn't do that; I had to eat to live. So I had to find a sane relationship with food. At that point in my life, therapy was inconceivable to me; even if I'd had the money, I didn't believe I deserved to be healed. I couldn't apply anything I'd learned from drying out in Guadalajara because I was a dry drunk; I'd simply stopped drinking cold turkey without examining any of the reasons why I'd ever started. I figured I'd just bushwhack my way into wellness.

Since one of the reasons I puked was to keep my weight under control, I first tried losing weight without puking. This led to fasting, which led to starving, which led to binging, which led to failure. Then I just tried to will myself to stop puking cold turkey. Failure. Fail enough times, and you lose your will to keep trying. Then it hit me: you teach what you have to learn. I was teaching my students to stay conscious, so that's where I would begin my own healing. Get quiet. Listen. Breathe. Tune inside and learn to ask questions that become steps. Could I stop puking? No. Could I control the amount I ate? No. What I could do was recognize that I had a problem, decide to do something about it, and stay conscious to the puking.

I decided that I would stay conscious throughout the puking process. That meant staying aware of whenever I felt I was being pulled into trance and not allowing myself to go numb. I made myself stop, breathe, and become aware of the way I frantically chewed my food, how I packed it all down, the process of puking it back up. I forced myself to stay present as a witness, feeling the disgust.

After I'd learned to become a witness, I found the courage to take another step. I was eating only one meal a day, but that meal would go on for hours upon hours. The next step was to limit my one gigantic meal to three hours, including breaks for puking. I could do that.

Next stage: *no matter what,* I wouldn't allow myself to throw up, even if it meant I got fat, which was an unspeakably horrid prospect for me; getting fat meant I'd be turning into my mother. And I did gain weight.

I stopped stepping on the scale after I hit 148 pounds, but I probably hit ten or fifteen pounds above that—a lot for my 5'7" frame. I still fell apart sometimes, but I got so I wasn't puking every day.

The next step was that I would limit my meal to just one plate of food, *no matter what*. It could be a platter heaped high, but just one plate. I still couldn't discern whether my stomach was full or empty, but limiting the amount of food on my plate would put a brake on eating to the point of explosion.

Slowly, very softly, but very clearly, my body began to speak to me during this process. It told me that I needed to take a closer look at my relationship with Ganga, which mirrored in some crucial ways what I'd endured in my relationship with my abusive mother. Ganga certainly was never violent, but like my mother, he was a consummate user. Like my mother, he exploited my own stupidity, ignorance, and naïveté. I didn't have enough self-esteem to stand up for myself; I didn't know how. I'd benefited from living at the Center for Yoga, traveling around the world with him on the book tour, and focusing so much on my Yoga practice. Ganga was a good playmate, taking me hiking, exposing me to new things. But my body told me that it was time to move on. For all the aspects of our time together that I treasured, most especially the book on double Yoga we'd created, it was clear that my relationship with Ganga was just another kind of orthodoxy: doing what someone else told me to do. It wasn't working for me to play by the strict rules of the Yoga orthodoxy, and it wasn't working for me to play by Ganga's rules either. I had to discover my own.

I started asking my body questions, and it started talking to me. It asked me for fish. That made no sense. I'd been a fanatic vegetarian for years; after all, the orthodoxy said that all good yogis and yoginis are vegetarian. But I prepared some fish. I ate it and sat there, the wide-eyed scientist, waiting to see the reaction. I was sure my stomach would hurl it. Instead, my body went, *Thank god.* This was something it could use. Then my body told me it wanted seaweed, nori mostly. It did not want grains. It was the beginning of a very slow process of learning what my body wanted. At first, it was hard to discern between the voice of my addictions and the voice of wisdom and healing. At least I was making new mistakes instead of the old ones. Step by painful step, I forged my unique path of healing.

I had learned that hunters would pray over the four-feet they killed. I was really enchanted with that. I'd come to see everything I ate as a kind of poison, so learning to pray over my food instead, to thank it for giving me its life force so that I could live, was radically important and healing for me. It helped me not to waste the food by puking it. Praying, giving thanks, was another way to choose life over and over again. I'd found an opening out of the maze, a way to heal myself. Years later, I saw a nutritionist to help me figure out what else I should be eating. When I moved onto an Indian reservation, I started eating game. But for now, I'd learned that the way to understand what I most needed to heal myself was to listen.

Bulimia is a behavior pattern that extends beyond food. I was bulimic with all sorts of things. I would gorge on information and puke it back up. Dive into something indiscriminately and just cut and run. I would approach everything with the attitude, *I can get through this. I can endure this.* The bulimics in my workshops do Yoga the same way: *Just let me push through this. I can take it.* The key to overcoming bulimic behavior—in fact, any addictive behavior—is to stop, breathe, feel, discover the real need, and then feed the true hunger inside.

Bulimia is the perfect example to illustrate that you can starve amid bounty. Let's work with how to listen to your body's deepest hungers and truly feed your starving Spirit. Accessing your intuition and practicing that level of discernment is crucial if you want to hear your body's wisdom.

SPIRITUAL FOCUS:
TUNING IN TO THE WISDOM OF YOUR BODY

Feeling your body can be an incredibly challenging step. Many of us have lost parts of ourselves by walling off something of great pain. That coping skill is often necessary to survive. But it's possible to reopen that chapter of life and distill the treasures from those intense times. Ten, twenty, thirty years later, I have been able to do healing around those times. I've been able to listen to and reclaim the person I called Annie the horse girl from those days. It took me a long time to access and consciously use the wisdom from Annie's life. I shut it all down with the pain and the addictions and the suicide attempts. Part of my healing has been going back to that part of my life to quest for the richness and the wisdom that came from that time, which I can now use every day. My suffering wasn't useless. Nor is yours; I want to teach you the wisdom of tuning in to your body and listening to its messages so that you too can reclaim your whole self.

WHAT ARE YOU HUNGRY FOR?

The slow, gradual process of healing my bulimia taught me the magnificence of listening to my body, feeding the hunger from within instead of numbing out to it. I learned to ask my inner wisdom better questions. For example: *What is it I really need right now? What can I do to fill my neediness even a little?* Those were questions I could begin to answer. I want to help you explore what you're truly longing for and how you can feed that soul-deep hunger—which usually has nothing whatsoever to do with food.

Most of our addictive behaviors come from an attempt (and failure) to feed our starved self. What do you crave? If you have a full-blown addiction—to food, alcohol, cigarettes, drugs—the truth is that the substance you crave will never meet the true yearning you have. The highest high only helps us forget the deeper yearning that seems impossible to deal with.

Take a closer look at your symptoms. Get curious. What's going on? *Why* do you have to smoke that pack of cigarettes? *Why* do you have to blow it out on the weekend? You feel hideous as a result and know you're destroying yourself, but it's supposedly giving you something. What deeper need is your addictive behavior trying to fill?

Get quiet, get grounded, and feel around inside. Many of my clients have developed deep cravings or addictions because they've cut themselves off from something they found meaningful for various reasons—they told themselves it wasn't practical, they couldn't make a living doing it, it wasn't something so-called good people or real grown-ups did, etc. Have you ever put away the things that delighted you—painting, running, weaving, dancing? Was there a moment when you declared, for example, *I'll never be a dancer, so therefore I won't dance*? See if you get a flash. Maybe you'll remember a moment when you put away that dream and took another route. It's not always wrong to take a different direction, but sometimes we turn away from something because we wrongly believe we have no other option. When that happens, we leak our soul's blood out of the hole left in us. Addictive behaviors are a destructive—and ineffective—way to try to fill that hole.

FEEDING A STARVING SELF

How can you begin to feed yourself when a destructive craving grabs you? The first step is always deep breathing because if you're trying to feed a starving self, what better way than to literally nourish the cellular tissue with life-giving oxygen? Already, miraculously, you will begin to feel more alive and restored.

Next ask your body: *What is it you're really needing right now?* Then do something that at least begins to touch that need. Doing something that stimulates your endorphins—the joy-producing chemicals in your brain—is always a good choice. What can you do right now that brings that shot of delight? Laugh? Sing? Dance?

So many of my clients crave chocolate. Ask yourself: *What do I really want here?* If the answer is that you want to bring sweetness into your life—sweetness with beneficial consequences—get creative. Ask your body what else would delight it. Sweet on the tongue is just one flavor to choose from. What else would feel sweet? Take a bath with wonderful oils that delight your nose. Get a massage. Smell a bouquet of flowers.

If you find yourself blindsided by an eating addiction, stop, breathe, and ask yourself, *Am I eating in a way that helps me become the person I most want to be, or am I eating to feed my addictions? Will eating this way brighten or dim my Spirit?*

How do you tell your Addict from your Spirit? When your Addict is talking, you'll feel a tightening in your belly or a feeling of sickness or nausea. That's a clue. It's hard to stay honest about this because we don't want to acknowledge those sensations, but can you be honest with yourself? Can you catch yourself about to respond in the usual way to that craving?

At those times when you feel dispirited or you're reaching those inevitable impasses, whether in Yoga or in daily life, ask yourself, *What can I do right now to triumph over my old behavior patterns?* In other words, disobey the commands of your old training and refocus on where you want to go on your life path instead of once again traveling into those old dimming, shaming places. This is an exercise in honoring the truth about yourself. The plethora of internal responses and options that will come up in answer to that question might surprise you. What you are really asking for is a new way. That frees the energy to move. Bringing that skillful awareness into your so-called ordinary moments can be exhilarating. This can be seriously fun! It's making a game of encouraging your consciousness to take a quantum leap.

Here's an example of catching a situation in daily life: you come home after a long, frustrating, hard day at work and go right to the refrigerator, pop a beer, and flop in front of the television. Your internal dialogue may be, *I'm exhausted. I need a break. I need to enjoy myself. I deserve this. I've earned it.* Two or four hours later, did you really deserve to give yourself that played-out feeling accompanied by a dull headache from the beer and television? Perhaps you could have served yourself better. How about a shower and half an hour of yoga? I've done both options in my life, and the latter wins hands-down every time! You'll feel great, awake, nourished, and proud of yourself instead of toxic and brain-dead. Ask yourself, *What is it I really need that I'm hoping beer and television/ice cream and cake/a cigarette and a cup of coffee will give me?*

Access your wisdom regarding actions and consequences. For example, binging leads to self-loathing, loss of self-respect, and degradation of your health. Get steady and ask yourself: *What do I really want?* If the answer is that you want to feel good, what else can you do that will result in that good feeling and also build your self-respect? Ask your body whether Yoga, taking a walk in nature, or putting on some music and dancing around your house would feed it. Do a dharma joust: what can you do instead in that moment that would actually make you feel good? Go listen to your favorite music. Turn the computer off and play with the kitty—immerse yourself in fur and purr.

Are you starved for touch, that most elemental of human connections? Most of us have a deficit here. Some of our neediness could go all the way back to a childhood in which our parents didn't understand the importance of touching and cuddling. We might seek to fulfill that need in damaging ways, for example, indiscriminate sex. Or maybe it goes the other way—we can't engage sexually with our mate because it's too charged, or we're alone and don't have a mate. If that's the case for you, pay for a quality massage. Can you include this as part of taking care of your needs? At the very least, you can massage your own hands and feet with a little oil, especially right before bedtime. Understand that touch is our most basic language. By receiving quality touch, our self-worth is steadied. Do you still greet your friends and loved ones with a hug? This is a good time to nourish yourself and them. Breathe and feel when you hug. Let that precious gift of affection soak into your cells. It's one of the most inexpensive ways to begin to fill that huge hole of need.

In the long term, create steps to help you find a way to develop your gifts, work with what delights you, and begin to flap the wings of your Spirit. One of my clients, Karl, was a commercial artist as well as a major overeater who'd developed diabetes. Eating sweets was poisonous to him, but he ate them constantly because he craved them constantly. I asked him: "How else can you create sweetness in your life?" Not in his marriage; it didn't feed him, it just supported him. Not in his work; he felt his commercial drawings were devoid of soul. I had him tune in and ask himself what he most craved. "I want to paint again" was the answer. I asked him to start doing just that. His canvases were huge—almost life size—realistic paintings of women in contemplation: passionate, beautiful, textured. They reminded me of Van Gogh. When Karl rediscovered his passion for painting, he lost his craving for the sweets that threatened his health.

So many of my clients have made life into an either-or proposition: *either I'm a breadwinner or an artist.* If you're a starving artist, it's time to find a way to incorporate creative expression back into your life. To be perfectly clear, go for *I am a breadwinner* and *an artist.*

Not sure what will feed you? Experiment! Go dancing Friday night, or sign up for a class. Check in with yourself. Have your destructive cravings waned? If so, you're on the way to feeding your starving soul.

DETOXIFY: WHAT FEEDS YOUR BRAIN

What do you feed your brain? I'm not talking about beer or sugar or chocolate—I'm talking about the ongoing gossip at the water fountain, bitching about the job or the wife or the husband. This is toxic stuff to pour into your head and cell tissue. What else feeds your insanity? How much time do you spend watching TV or reading magazines that put inhumanity and ugliness front and center? I've learned the hard way that I have to be vigilant so my mind doesn't become a toxic dumping ground. Even movies I enjoy give me a hideous headache the next day— is that worth it?

Screening out this toxicity is central to keeping my Spirit bright. When there's too much noise in my head, it's impossible to tune in to my needs. I don't watch the news if I can help it. I don't read daily newspapers. I don't watch TV. I may not be up on the latest headlines, but I always manage to find a way to learn what I need to know. I may not know who the hottest contestants are on *American Idol* or *Top Chef*— or even much beyond that these shows exist (my cowriter told me about them), but it hasn't stopped me from enjoying the true cultural treasures around me—music, art, Cirque du Soleil. I want to feed myself the best of what we aspire to, not the lowest common denominator.

The ongoing complaining, gossiping, filth-spreading energy—does that brighten or dim your Spirit? If you're having a good gossip, the energy will feel bright, but afterward you'll get a bitterness seeping into your heart and mind, like when you drink too much coffee. The more we indulge in toxic behavior, the farther we drive our Spirit out, leaving us spiritually bereft; we starve our souls in the midst of plenty.

PHYSICAL FOCUS:
NOURISHING BODY AND SOUL

Yoga poses can do so much to help you build discernment and awareness, and they help you get quiet enough to hear what your body and intuition are telling you.

POSES TO PINPOINT THE HUNGER WITHIN

If you're having trouble identifying what you're truly hungering for, certain still poses can be very helpful. Breathe into the part of your body where you're feeling the hunger, that is, your belly. Abdominal poses are great for that. Or if it is hunger for love, breathe into your heart. I recommend Chest Opener on the Wall (see page 92), Camel (see page 30), Warrior I (see page 61), or Wheel (see page 157). Move deeply into these poses for five to ten breaths while asking yourself, *What do I really want right at this moment?* Listen for your body's response.

POSES THAT INCREASE AWARENESS

Certain Yoga poses specifically increase awareness. The second chakra bears the lessons of the intestine: the ability to discern what nourishes you and what doesn't. The Forrest Yoga Basic Moves described in chapter one; abdominals such as Elbow to Knee, Abs with a Roll, and Frog Lifting Through; as well as new poses listed here such as Bridge with a Roll and Dolphin all increase the intelligence in the second chakra.

Here is a sequence that includes them all. Some have been described in previous chapters, while others are new and their explanations follow. Doing poses in this sequence will be safe and healing for your body and will amp up your awareness big time.

POSE	PAGE	HOLD TIME/REPETITIONS
Cross-Legged Side Bend	61	5 breaths
Abs with a Roll	59	3–5 rounds
Frog Lifting Through	59	3–5 rounds
Bridge with a Roll	155	10 breaths
Dolphin	156	10 breaths
Sun Salutations	223	10 rounds

In the last round, instead of stepping into Lunge, step into Warrior I (see p. 61) and hold for 5 breaths.

Cobra over a Roll	156	5–10 breaths
Camel	30	5 breaths
Wheel	157	3–5 rounds
Elbow to Knee	58	6 rounds
(with one leg straight)		

POSE	PAGE	HOLD TIME/REPETITIONS
Cross-Legged Twist	158	3–5 breaths
Back Release Pose	159	5 breaths
Neck Release Pose	64	5 breaths
Savasana	159	5 minutes

SIDE BEND IN BADDHA KONASANA WITH TWO ARM POSITIONS

Side Bend in Baddha Konasana with Two Arm Positions stretches the hips, the lungs and opens up the lymph nodes. Deep breaths cleanse the lymph glands and clarify perception.

Sit in Baddha Konasana, soles of the feet together, and active. Place your left hand straight out from the left hip, resting on the fingertips. First arm position: inhale, lift the right arm up. Exhale, relax the neck to the left, leaning your left ear toward the left shoulder, bending the left elbow, pressing the palm of the left hand down. With your right arm extended past your right ear, reach to the left, keeping both hands ac-

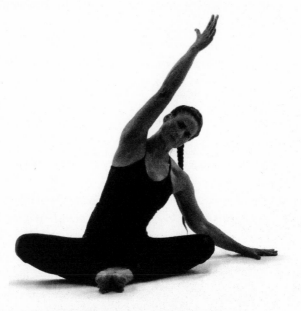

Side Bend in Baddha Konasana with Two Arm Positions

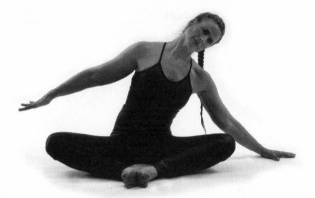

tive. Move the left shoulder away from the left ear. Breathe through your whole right side, washing your breath through your lymph glands in the armpit, through the right ribs and the right side of the waist, down into the lymph glands in the right inner groin. Stay for three to five breaths, stretching the breath and intercostal muscles.

Second arm position: stretch the right arm out to the right with your fingertips twelve inches from the floor, feeling with the arm for the angle that stretches the right side of the neck and the right upper trapezius. Stay for three to five breaths.

To come out of the pose, leave the neck relaxed to the left and reach your right arm to the right to pull your torso upright. Leaving the neck relaxed, use the left hand to pick the head up. Repeat on the other side.

BRIDGE WITH A ROLL

Bridge with a Roll, a variation of Bridge (see page 60), will turn on your inner leg muscles to support you in Wheel. Place a roll between your legs and lie on your back, knees bent and feet flat on the floor about a foot apart, with your heels aligned below your knees. Exhale and tilt your tailbone up. Squeeze the roll between your legs and lift the pelvis and torso up, keeping your shoulders, neck, and head on the floor. Inhale and telescope the ribs toward your face. Exhale, press through your feet, and tilt your tailbone up even more; keep squeezing the roll. Take five to eight deep breaths. Keep your tailbone tucked as you come out of the pose. Remove the roll once you are all the way down.

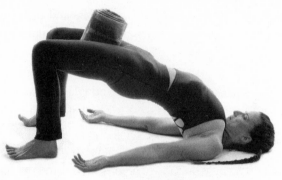

Bridge with a Roll

DOLPHIN

Dolphin is a real power pose. Move onto your forearms and knees. Grasp your upper arms to measure the proper elbow distance, and then bring your forearms out so they're parallel. Exhale, curl your toes under, and straighten your legs. Hold for ten breaths.

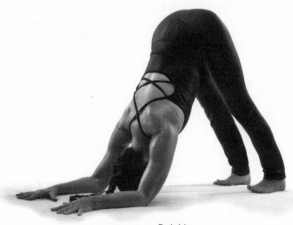

Dolphin

COBRA OVER A ROLL

Cobra over a Roll gets right into the belly of the beast, exorcising the little demons that might be in there. Grab your roll and lie with your belly on top of it at the navel. Take three deep breaths lying down on the roll, allowing it to massage the knots in the belly and intestines. To come into

Cobra, place your elbows under the shoulders and tuck your tailbone down toward the floor, squeezing your knees and anklebones together. Get your feet active. Inhale and move up into Cobra, lifting your elbows three inches off the floor and telescoping your ribs forward. Exhale, sliding the shoulder blades down the back and relaxing the belly onto the roll to decompress the lower back. On each inhale, pull the ribs forward, teaching the mid and upper back to arch as the lower back learns to lengthen. Hold Cobra for five to ten breaths, keeping the neck relaxed. To come out of the pose, keep the tailbone tucked and the ribs telescoping forward as you lower all the way down.

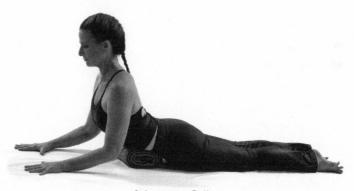

Cobra over a Roll

WHEEL

Do the sequence on page 153 to warm up safely for Wheel. Wheel is a powerful, exhilarating, deep back-bending pose! Begin in Bridge (see page 60). Place your hands under your shoulders, fingers pointing toward your heels, exhale, and press up powerfully! Lower the top rim of your sacrum an inch toward the floor, tilt your tailbone up toward the ceiling, and telescope your ribs away from the lower back. Press strongly through your legs while keeping your feet active and your neck relaxed. To come out of the pose, come back into Bridge first, and then come out of Bridge. Repeat Wheel three to five times.

If Wheel is not your pose for today, do Camel (see page 30) two more times.

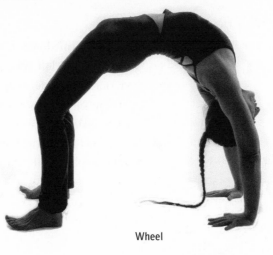

Wheel

CROSS-LEGGED TWIST

Cross-Legged Twist gets mobility in the spine and moves some of the numbness out of the brain and butt. Twists wring out tension in your upper, mid, and lower back as well as the organs.

Sit cross-legged, put your left hand on your right knee, and your right hand either on the floor behind your pelvis or behind your back to hold your left thigh or grab your waistband. Inhale lifting up through the spine and chest, using the arms as leverage. Exhale. Keep lifting while twisting. Take three to five breaths and change sides.

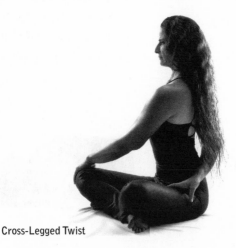

Cross-Legged Twist

BACK RELEASE POSE

Back Release pose is great to let your back warm down. Lie on your back. Bend your knees, feet on the floor. Bring the left ankle on top of the right thigh, letting the left knee open out to the side. Keep both feet active while inhaling and lifting the legs up off the floor. Exhale and thread your left arm through your left leg, your right arm around the outside of your right thigh, clasping the hands at the right shin or the back of the right thigh. Stay for five breaths. Repeat on the other side.

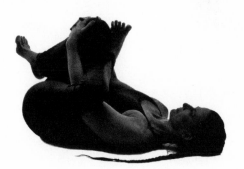

Back Release Pose

SAVASANA

Savasana, or Corpse pose, is a quiet time to let the wonderful new energy from your practice soak in to the cell tissue. Lie down on your back with your spine straight, hands and feet flopped out to the sides. Slide the shoulder blades down the spine, pulling the shoulders away from the neck. Tuck the tailbone down and relax your lower back. Breathe deeply for five minutes.

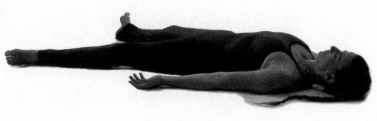

Savasana

Are you ready to stop starving amid plenty? Are you ready to pay attention to those hunger pains that are your body's deepest wisdom? When you begin to listen, truly listen, to your intuition, you'll find the strength to stop following any authority that speaks against your heart and Spirit. You'll disobey the dictates of your addictions. That's thrilling! You'll walk yourself into a world that's far more compelling.

7

WALKING THE GOOD RED ROAD:
BECOMING A HEALER

THE FLYER was for a workshop called Indian Summer. The teacher, a psychic healer named the Reverend Rosalyn Bruyere, a Medicine Woman of the Hopi, Navajo, and Cree nations, promised to teach healing arts from a Native American perspective. As I held the paper in my hand, a longing from two decades earlier stirred in me.

As a kid, I'd discovered that my kinship wasn't with people; it was with wind, earth, animals, stars, fire, lightning, thunder, storms. I used to wander up into the San Gabriel mountains above Glendora where long ago the Tongva Indians had made their home among the rocky earth and high chaparral. I'd move in silence, as if I could hear their traditions calling to me. I'd do my best to do whatever I thought an Indian would do—track the raccoons, coyotes, kit foxes, and wildcats; try to disappear inside the bark of a pine, oak, or juniper; forage for edibles like prickly pear.

I longed for the deep connection to earth that Native Americans seemed to have. Whenever I read about the plight of the Indians—driven from their land, stripped of their culture—it made my heart bleed. Tribe after tribe: extinct. My own life at the time felt equally withered and pointless; it was just like me to yearn for something that was pretty much dead and gone.

Twenty years later, I was in Los Angeles. I'd left Ganga and opened my first studio, which I fittingly called The Turning Point. While I might have put my Orthodox Yoga phase behind me—my whole life has been about stepping outside of the orthodox—I was still thirsting for someone to mentor me in my quest to become a healer. Perhaps studying with Rosalyn would direct my own powers of healing and walk me into magic. I signed up for the workshop.

When Rosalyn took the stage on the first day of class at the Healing Light Center, she just about knocked me out of my chair. You couldn't have ordered up anyone more tailor-made to challenge all my prejudices. Here was this broad done up in full makeup with fake eyelashes, pointy heels, carrying around about eighty extra pounds of fat. It was impossible not to think about my mother. Yet from the moment she opened her mouth to speak, Rosalyn was funny as hell, compelling, provocative, seductive.

I'd found the medium for my magic.

Rosalyn commanded the stage on her tippy, gold, lame high heels. She captivated us all with her lectures on medicine wheels and other aspects of Native American healing, and the power of storms, lightning, floods, earthquakes—the same abundant, chaotic manifestations of energy I'd always been drawn to. Having learned many of her teachings from Navajo elders, she taught us about mediumship, hands-on healing, and chelation—running energy in certain patterns to pull out the toxicity within a person's body. She taught us how to feel where energy was stuck, pooled, or off in some way and how to help it flow freely again by drawing energy from the earth, running it through our hearts, and out through our hands.

Half the time in class, I was so electrified by what I was experiencing that the hair stood up on the nape of my neck; half the time my skin was crawling because I couldn't stand the other students around me. The workshop was a magnet for all these askew people: a lot of abused women, a whole lot of whackaberry cranks spouting airy-fairy New Age crap. One guy sidled up to me and announced, "We were lovers in a previous life." That's a real winning line, right up there with "Come up and see my etchings." I was so allergic to all that stuff. As a Yoga teacher, I worked and lived in this very strange New Age market filled with so many deceptive promises that I was embarrassed to be associated with it; I was afraid that anything I put out into the world would end up on the same nonnutritive shelf. I call that sweet sickening process spiritual diabetes.

But Rosalyn seemed to have her own internal bullshit detector. She'd sweep away the vogues of the moment: "Affirmations are like whipped cream on garbage," she told us. "You can make it sweet, but it's still garbage." But she also had powers I couldn't deny, though I wanted to. When Rosalyn channeled what she called disincarnate beings, she didn't just imitate, say, an ancient Chinese man. Damn if this Valley Mom didn't *become* him in voice and body language through a transformation I couldn't begin to fathom. Was she just a drama queen or a great actress? If it was a scam, it was a pretty elaborate one. She kept poking at my doubts, declaring, "This isn't about whether mediumship exists. If that's still a question for you, you don't show up at this workshop. That mind is not welcome in the workshop. This is about how to work as a medium."

Being a medium didn't appeal to me; I didn't like the idea of moving aside so someone else could come in. But when Rosalyn started lecturing on sensing energy, my ears pricked up. Again, though, I was distracted by all the whackaberries rhapsodizing about the sweeping, swooshing whatevers they were seeing. "Oh, look, I see unicorns! And rainbows! Isn't it amazing?" I wasn't seeing anything. Were these people delusional liars, or was I so head-blind I couldn't get out of my own way? It was a period of intense self-doubt and doubting those around me (with very good reasons!).

Then I decided that seeing other people's energy was a capacity that we all have, just as we all have eyes. I had the potential to see energy, but my seeing skills were like an atrophied muscle. Bingo! I knew what to do with an atrophied muscle. You need to work it at the rate it will respond.

I made up something I called the Seeing Game. I started by looking at something, then looking away, then back again to see what I'd missed. I began to see that whatever I looked at emitted something, like a disturbance in the air; I realized that was energy. Wherever the energy would have the most activity would show the most agitation. By choosing to look for it, I got better at spotting it.

I became willing to attempt to train beyond my eyes—to take information in whatever way it arrived. Smells in particular gave me a lot of information. When the body isn't quite right, there's a weirdness to its smell. It took me a while to decode these signals. I'd check with people to ask them how they were feeling. Eventually I figured out that a dehydrated man smells like cat piss. Women with fibroids have a particular scent. If someone had a metallic smell, I started wondering whether he had a problem with some internal organ or was detoxing drugs.

When I first started practicing running energy I wasn't sure I was feeling it, but then I started hunting for the signals. Soon I could sense almost a magnetic pull. Stuck energy feels like mud or a blood clot; it's an eddy instead of a stream. Sometimes I'd feel a hot spot, almost like a solar flare, beneath my hand; the corralled energy reminded me of a horse stuck in a box canyon. Other times energy felt like a black hole; no matter how hard I tried, I couldn't fill that sinkhole. This is another type of signal. But then there were times when I'd try to put energy into someone's body, only to feel energy pushing back, as if the body was saying, *I can't eat any more. I'm full.*

I'd start by tuning in on someone and just notice what sensations I was picking up. Everything emits energy. I'd scan someone and see what parts of her body were emitting energy in an aberrant way. Dim, dull energy felt like an actual roadblock. A nauseous feeling in my gut told me someone was dealing with what I took to calling emotional pus balls, painful feelings archived in the tissue. I'd zero in on which area to work with, feeling, listening, smelling for the next trail. My hands might want to go with someone's neck, even if I experienced a nauseous or choking sensation. I wasn't thinking so much as I was intuiting or empathing.

I experimented with how to work with each of these energies. If I felt that solar flare, I needed to open up the area around it so the energy could disperse. With a sinkhole, I needed to create a catchment system so the energy could pool, just as a flash flood in the desert needs to be able to sit for a while before it can soak in. Slowly I developed a personal vocabulary of healing. Women with osteoporosis had sinkholes. Cancer looked like a teeming pool of churning maggots, a ravenous beast devouring its host. Bone is slow; the nervous system is a big electrical *whoosh!* of energy.

I began talking with the people I was running energy on, poking around for an explanation of the dissonance I was feeling. Someone might tell me about a neck injury, but the real story was that she'd had a car crash with her kids in the car—she'd been terribly frightened because she hadn't been able to use her mama bear energy to protect them. My healing had to go beyond massaging bone and muscles; I had to help free the energy that was stuck there because of the psychic trauma. Pain often has a deeper story; when I excavated the story, I could be more effective in healing the pain.

I still couldn't turn off that chattering voice of negativity inside my head—*You're delusional; you're crazy*—but I also couldn't deny that I was helping people heal. I'd work on them, and they would tell me how much better they felt. Still, I struggled with my own desire to be a healer.

While I felt I was making great progress as a healing student, something was missing from my life. I began to admit to myself that I was lonely. I didn't just want a replacement for Ganga to fill my bed; I wanted a true partner, someone who could share in my mission for healing others. One night I dreamed of eagles. Eagles have always been wake-up calls for me. Whenever you see one, stop whatever you're doing and pay attention! The eagle flies highest, is the messenger of the gods. In my dream, two eagles were climbing up a shaft of wind, doing these incredible acrobatics. They seemed to be fighting, tangling at the crest of their flight, and then tumbling downward and flying apart. Over and over and over. When I woke from the dream, I felt I'd been given an important piece of information, but I didn't know what to do with it.

Months later I happened to see a documentary on eagles. The pair in my dream weren't fighting; they were mating! Something clicked into place. I'd been calling for a mate in the best way I knew how—just putting the energy out into the universe. *Come to me! I'm waiting!* The dream was telling me something about that. Shortly afterward, a friend told me, "I want you to meet this man. He's an artist, and his name is Heyoka. Here's his portfolio." On the cover was a photo of one of Heyoka

Merrifield's sculptures: a magnificent carving of a man with powerful wings and the head of an eagle with piercing eyes. My eagle man. It gave me the shivers.

When Heyoka, a wiry Cherokee man with quiet, deep-set eyes like a deer and long brown hair shot with silver, arrived to pick up his portfolio, he unrolled a length of velvet to show me the exquisite jewelry he made from gold, silver, turquoise, and pipestone. The craftsmanship and level of detail were stunning, but that's not what caught my attention. The pieces were radiating pure, bright energy. "What did you do to these?" I asked him. Surprised, Heyoka explained that he did ceremony over them, awakening the energy in the stones, metals, and archetypal symbols so they'd become shields for the wearers.

In that instant we made a magical connection, not just as future lovers, but as a practiced magic worker with a potential apprentice. Heyoka fixed those deep-set eyes on me. "I have to drive north. Come with me." I jumped into his van, and we went to visit a camp in Nevada City led by Hyemeyohsts Storm, the same Medicine Man who'd trained Rosalyn—another magical connection. The camp was enchanting—people of all different races and colors and sizes doing art and medicine work and living together. The main meeting place was called Phoenix Lodge, which got my attention; I was looking to rise from the ashes of my life too. For the first time, I watched Heyoka go into ceremony. I met his family too. In my time there, I became convinced that this way of life was next on my path as a healer. It was as if everything Rosalyn had been teaching us came alive. These weren't dead Indians; they were living and practicing everything I'd just been learning about and more.

The universe has its own timing. I made a phone call and discovered that my studio, The Turning Point, had lost its lease. I took it as another sign to jump—move in with Heyoka on his land up in Washington State and study what the Native Americans call the Red Road: the way of good medicine and healing.

With my typical flare for planning, I tossed everything I owned into my Subaru Brat—was there ever a more perfectly named car for me?—with the trailer and headed north with a map Heyoka had sent me. Up in Washington, the temperature plummeted, and there I was in shorts and a crop top, literally out of my element. When I got off the ferry across the Columbia River and checked the map for directions, I discovered that every road marked on it was called Primitive Road—thank you, U.S. Government. Lost and freezing, I drove aimlessly for hours as night fell. Finally I approached a huge gray hump that looked like nothing more than a brontosaurus's butt. It was an earth shelter—a house that is made to be underground, covered with earth—that Heyoka was in the middle of building. Shivering down to my bones, I stumbled inside what would become my home for the next five and a half years.

The next morning I woke up and wandered outside to find Heyoka digging holes around the sweat lodge and then putting a whole fish and a corn kernel into each one, just the way I'd read about Indians planting crops. Another sign that the Indians weren't dead. I felt a rush of hope. They'd found a way to survive, and so would I.

At first I was very lonely. Heyoka lived in near isolation on his forty acres, and most of his time was consumed with the process of sacred jewelry making. We barely interacted with other members of the tribe. I slowly figured out how to make myself useful. I learned how to chop wood and carry water, how to use buffing tools and a blowtorch to assist in creating the artwork. Once in a while, I would go do a workshop to make money. Sometimes I would teach Yoga to people who showed up for medicine.

Then I learned to bead. I created beautiful, intricate beading on Heyoka's shirts to wear while he sold his art. I'd never made artwork before, and I loved it. But the process was new for me. All the skills I'd acquired up to then—training horses, teaching Yoga—had no clear ending. Heyoka had to teach me when a work of art is done. I learned how to make an art piece that had a beginning, middle, and end. I discovered I had a great sense for putting colors together. Soon people were asking me to bead for them. I'd pray and ask for a vision of what the art should look like and the energy it needed to contain that would work best for the individual. Beading was such an act of will and strain, it helped me focus. My days were spent beading, doing Yoga, helping in the art studio, cooking, cleaning. But my most important occupation became learning through osmosis what Heyoka had to teach me about Spirit.

Heyoka lived a life of Spirit. He'd taken the name Heyoka because it means "Sacred Clown"—someone whose role is sometimes to mock or imitate people in order to show them that their pain is pointless. A master craftsman, he's what's known as a Shield Maker; he sees his mission as creating not merely jewelry, but awakened pieces of medicine that provide blessings, protection, and a mirror for the people who wear them. For him, prayer is an essential part of his creation. I'd watch Heyoka go into ceremony to pray over every aspect of his process, from blessing his tools and workspace at the beginning of every day to blessing each piece upon completion. He would cleanse the room with sage smoke, washing himself in the process, setting his intent, clearing out whatever energy didn't serve. He used both incredible precision and his deepest intuition in creating his jewelry.

When he was done with something, we'd take it into this hidden room behind a tapestry, his *kiva*—a sacred space of the Southwest Indians—where we would do an Awakening and Blessing of the Shield ceremony. Filling his pipe with tobacco, Heyoka would first call in the energy and the protective powers of the Four Directions, then the elements and the planets. Then he would call in White Buffalo Calf Woman, the powerful spirit of the woman who first came to the Lakota and gave them their seven ceremonies, including sweat lodge and pipe, to help them become spiritually rich again. He'd pray that whatever person was attracted to the piece of jewelry he'd made would benefit from its special energy and protection from malicious powers, that Beauty would soak into them, that they would learn to embody it. He prayed to send Beauty and magic and balance into the world through his art.

Watching Heyoka pray was a revelation. I'd gone to church with my Catholic friend Annette once, but I can remember praying only once when I was young. As I described earlier, my brother suffered a great deal from his obesity. I wanted to take the burden off of him and put it onto me, so I sneaked out to the backyard and directed my words to where I figured heaven would be. *If you're really there, God, then let me take this off of him.* I wasn't much surprised when I got no answer. When Heyoka saw how much I craved to learn ceremony, he invited me into the process. I began to see the power and mystery of prayer and how effective it can be when done properly.

Tobacco is central to the pipe ceremony. Heyoka started teaching me ceremony using cigarettes because that made sense for me, although I also found it hysterically funny because tobacco reminded me of Maya, my original Truth Speaker. One day I was working in a Santa Fe market, helping Heyoka sell his jewelry, when I met two women and ended up doing a healing ceremony on them. One of them gave me a pipe as thanks. I had been dreaming about my pipe for months before this happened. The bowl was beautiful, made out of pipestone, or catlinite. I wasn't sure I deserved it. Heyoka wasn't sure if I was ready yet, but he directed me how to carve it down to fit my mouth and then taught me how to use it.

Over the years, I learned how to be a Medicine Person, a healer, and a Pipe Carrier—someone who has taken on the responsibility for the health and well-being of the people. It's much like being a rabbi; I'm responsible for teaching the people in my tribe, but what they do with the teachings is up to them. As I see it, as a Pipe Carrier, I renew the web of mystery and magic each time I bring out the pipe.

I first learned to pray by calling in a whole group of folks I call the Supernaturals, or the Sacred Ones—Thunderbird, Sisiutl, the spirit or intelligence of the wind kachina. The pipe helped me connect to the Sacred Ones. It helped me focus on whoever had asked me to do ceremony or prayers or healing. If someone was in the hospital, I might pray for their pain to ease and their healing to quicken. I started actively praying for the children in the world. This was a huge act of courage for me—overcoming the exhausting apathy of *I can't really make a difference in this world.*

Whenever a Pipe Carrier smokes a pipe, she smokes it for the people, including herself. That meant I had to do prayers for myself, and that was a really hard step for me. I could pray for the land, the water, the humans, the deer folk—but it was very difficult to figure out what to say for myself, or to feel that I deserved to be able to ask. I prayed for a long time for the Sacred Ones to talk to me in a way I could understand.

Despite my role as a Pipe Carrier, I struggled for acceptance in the tribe. I was terribly shy, afraid of doing something sacrilegious, but my desire to learn kept pushing me forward. I did a Sun Dance, a ceremony of purification and rebirth, before I was formally accepted. This disobedience led me to recognize that there was something greater than me to put my trust and faith in, and it gave me permission to go farther. This opening led to a profound vision. I have since been taken in and prayed for by many different tribes, and I am really grateful for it.

One day I was sitting with my pipe by the Columbia River, looking down at the water rushing over the round river rocks. My head throbbed from a migraine. I was fasting from food and water, which is traditional. I worried about stressing my body so much that I would bring on an epileptic fit. Maybe I was just too toxic for the Sacred Ones to bother with. Heyoka had always prayed so respectfully, but in my state of mind, all I could manage was: "Sacred Ones, what the fuck am I doing here?"

You know how the air feels different when there's a rainbow or lightning or the aurora borealis? Suddenly I could feel the opening of gates. I got quiet and stopped my growly energy long enough to feel the shift. My hair was standing on end. I scanned the rocks for predators. Rattlesnakes? Lynx? Cougar? Bear? Then up, over the river, I saw a vision. It was me, a gigantic me, standing, arms outstretched, hair down. My feet were planted in the earth, rainbows were radiating from my hands and feet, criss-crossing around the planet and back through my legs and through and around my body. I was surrounded by the sun and moon and stars. I was afraid to look away, but I also wanted the vision to go away. *You are delusional,* a voice inside me said, but I told it to shut the fuck up. In that moment I felt the wall of ice around my heart breaking. My heart surged, even though it was brittle and I feared it couldn't stretch without shattering. I allowed myself to truly feel my deepest desire—to be able to do something good in the world, whatever that was.

I turned a little toward it, glancing at it from the corner of my eye. Rustling around in my tobacco bag, I refilled my pipe and lit it. "Sacred Ones, that's really beautiful—what the *fuck* does that mean?" I didn't get a direct answer, but something in me changed in that moment. I felt how big I actually was compared to how I'd seen myself before—this little piece of trash struggling to do good things. I'd believed that I could wipe my slate clean only by working myself to death. Now I felt there was something mysterious, something magnificent, inside me. What I was seeing was an invitation from the Sacred Ones to accept and move into doing my part in healing the world. In the days and years to come, I would backslide into despair many times, but now I knew this unshakable truth to be within me.

It took me years and a lot of experimenting to clarify the meaning of that vision. I began to read about Black Elk, a healer and Medicine Man of the Oglala Lakota (Sioux). He's best known for sharing the teachings of the Sioux with a white man named John Neihardt (who earned the name Flaming Rainbow), who published them as *Black Elk Speaks.* In that book he shared a powerful vision he'd received through a "rainbow door" when he was nine years old, about his mission to protect a "hoop of peoples" around a sacred tree on the "good red road" that is the true good medicine of the native peoples. At the time Black Elk had his vision, the assault on the traditions of the Sioux was well under way; their culture and Spirit were dying out. Black Elk proclaimed, "The Rainbow Hoop of the People has been broken." He wanted to restore it, and this became his life's work. He'd prayed "that the sacred tree might bloom again and the people find their way back to the sacred hoop and the good red road. . . . O, make my people live!"

When you walk the red road, you choose to walk with an honoring and awareness of the laws of medicine and nature. It means that you feel the sky, the earth. You're aware of the energy around you. You're open to the Beauty in the world and choose to consciously embody Beauty as you move through life.

Reading about Black Elk's life's work helped me to articulate my own—I call it Mending the Rainbow Hoop of the People. I love playing in the Great Mystery of life and creation. I love that my mission is growing and evolving with such sweetness.

BECOMING YOUR OWN HEALER

Part of my mission in Mending the Hoop of the People is to teach others to become healers. I believe that we can all develop our intuition to help heal ourselves and others. One of the things I prized about my years on the reservation was seeing the initiation ceremonies the people used to hone intuition and the skillfulness in wielding it. Children who grow up with Native American traditions see the importance of developing these skills, of becoming aware of the sensitive, magical part of ourselves that don't yet have outlets. Western culture squashes and invalidates our nature so we don't develop our intuition, nor do we know how to use the information from our intuition as a tool for improving the quality of our daily life. I am working to correct that.

I've learned to view the human as an awesome mystery encased in skin. We need to develop the utmost respect for that human mystery, and we do so when we begin to move the energy inside the body.

Heyoka taught me that prayer is a beautiful and powerful tool to help listen within and without. I've learned through trial and error how to pray in the most effective way for myself. When it comes to working with intuition and healing, check out what feels true to you. Be your own authority, and learn to develop your own truth shield. At first, you'll be feeling around and flailing. Sure, you'll screw up. So what? That's how you learn.

SPIRITUAL FOCUS:
SEEING ENERGY AND EMPATHING

I now teach my students the Seeing Game that I made up as a child and evolved in Rosalyn Bruyere's class and beyond. It helps you hone the skill of becoming more aware of what's right in front of you. Improving the quality of your perceiving opens you up to the wonders of the world you live in and deepens your wisdom.

We constantly filter what's around us so we can function in the world. If I'm tracking, I'm looking for footprints, not at the stars or the sky. We're so focused on getting to work or the store that we close out a huge percentage of the magical cosmos. Sometimes we need to look up, as I learned in the Himalayas in Nepal at sunrise. I had to look above the cloud layers to see the tops of the Himalayas kissed by first light.

The first part of the Seeing Game is to look around. Then close your eyes and re-create your surroundings in as much detail as possible. Now open your eyes and look around again. What did you miss? Now really study what's in your line of vision, down to the greatest detail. When you walk into a room, make a game out of noticing everything you can. This trains your brain to bring in more information. Be playful; entice your intuition out of hiding.

Now deepen the exercise by practicing seeing energy. This isn't some esoteric skill that only psychics possess. We all know how to see and feel energy already. Walk into work and notice what kind of mood your boss is in. How did you pick that up? You did this by reading energy, body language, posture, tone of voice, breathing, and so on. Each of us has the potential to see intuitively; we just don't actively practice this skill in our daily lives. However, just like any other muscle, we can set about awakening and exercising these atrophied seeing muscles.

Start by quieting your mind, body, and energy by breathing deeply. Now look at someone. Notice where your eyes are drawn. Trust this information and look more closely to where your eyes focus. What do you see? Does that area of his body look darker or brighter compared to the areas around it? Does the energy feel constricted or rigid there? If you're working with a friend, you can ask for confirmation of what you sense. In any case, practice looking at people from an overall energetic perspective—the general vibe you pick up—as well as a more specific physical area.

Now practice empathing, the process by which you feel what someone else is feeling. Feel what happens in your own body when you are near someone who is nervous or scared. What do you feel and where? What's your reaction? Does your stomach tighten or do you stop breathing? Feel what happens in your own body when you're near someone unhappy or angry as opposed to someone who is happy and bubbly. How does your own body and energy shift in her presence?

As with seeing energy, it's important to quiet your own vibe and change from thinking to perceiving and feeling so that you can tune in to the more subtle signals your body may be picking up from the people around you. As you link up with another person's breath, energy, or vibe, what are you feeling in your body and where? If you're working with a friend, share your experiences to find out if you felt what he felt; this will help you fine-tune your information. As you begin to feel (empath), play with moving those feelings through your own body. Experiment . . . what worked in you? Then ask your friend to do the same thing you did that was successful in moving the energy. Track the results.

When you're beginning to empath, it's very common to be drawn to areas where you have had issues. For example, if you're shut down in your pelvic area because of some past trauma, you may feel that the other person's pelvic area is shut down, rigid, or shielded—or that her neck and throat areas are blocked. If you've dealt with similar issues or areas in your own body, your past behavioral issues (the ones that you have worked through) become your allies because you can recognize them in others. However, if you don't know your own stuff, you're going to get hooked and triggered by the other person. For example, if you are or were bulimic, you may feel like puking. Don't blame your reaction on the person you're working with. Go after these unrevealed areas of yourself and examine your own patterns and dynamics; please work with a qualified psychotherapist if necessary. This is an opportunity to learn a way to unwind and work through the pattern. You may then be able to help others with the same pattern, if you choose.

When I do my teacher training Yoga ceremonies, I help my trainees work with empathing and seeing with an exercise called Seeing Circle. All the trainees sit in a circle. A trainee volunteers to step into the middle of the circle and goes into a pose, which makes it easier for others to sense her energy. Each trainee in turn reports what he sees: "I'm noticing a tightness here, a wide open face, lots of energy in the arms, a dead butt." The trainees take turns testing out their intuitive flashes: Are they picking up tension in her neck or jaw? Are there areas of her body where the energy feels brighter or darker—or stuck? Do they sense hot spots or black holes? The student in the pose confirms the correct suppositions so the trainees can hone in more closely. Suppose her chest feels dark. What could be going on? Is there a story there? Working together, they might determine that she has a tender heart because of, say, a painful romantic experience, so she's collapsed around it, suffocating her chest area in an effort to protect herself. We would then work with her to bring breath into the area and watch/feel the energy rise there while encouraging her to change her pose so that she can physiologically create more space there. Bringing new feeling and breath into an area where old feelings have been trapped opens the door to releasing old feelings and stories.

This exercise is effective because the trainees learning to empath get direct feedback about whether or not they're on track. What's most important is not to edit what comes up for you as you explore empathing another person. It can take a while to develop real discernment and skill, or to separate what you're genuinely picking up from someone else's energy as opposed to projecting your own experience. This can also be an intensely emotional experience for the healer as the student's trapped emotions erupt to the surface. If working with a human is too difficult, practice seeing energy on a plant or your pet—you need to practice these skills a lot. Empathing makes you a more sensitive, informed person as you take in truths based on your body's wisdom.

INTUITION IN YOUR DAILY LIFE

You can also strengthen your intuition by road-testing it daily. The next time you're in the middle of one of those life situations that send you into a tailspin, pause, take a breath, and in the middle of that whirlwind, ask internally, *What does my intuition tell me about this situation?* By taking that moment to get still, to ask, and to listen, you invite your intuition to participate in your daily life. Your intuition and internal body signals will speak to you frequently if you listen. Just as you give up speaking or trying to communicate when someone doesn't listen to you, your intuition's voice gets fainter and then falls silent when you don't listen to it. When we begin to work with our intuitive flashes, we open to wonder and possibility, and our life can regain the sparkly magical quality that faded so long ago or perhaps never had a chance to shine.

Forrest Yoga is all about finding out what is happening *right now* and responding to that. How do you begin to honor and heal yourself? By paying attention to what is going on inside and outside of you, and primarily by seeing what is not honoring you. How do you feel inside emotionally? Physically? How do you talk to yourself? Honing your intuition, you can begin to recognize the undermining behavioral patterns that are a subtle act of aggression against yourself, reframe them, and make a more healing choice.

THE POWER OF PRAYER

Prayer connects your mind and Spirit to a bigger place, from which you can assess an issue. I pray when I need to get into that more connected place. Prayer helps me listen deeply inside and outside. Even if I don't get answers, I appreciate the deep silence. When I come into a sacred space to pray, whether sitting on my mat or with my pipe, it's incredible to feel that I'm part of the sacred—and therefore I am also sacred. I need to reconnect with the truth of that on a regular basis.

Prayer is also a way to give some sacred time to what's uppermost in your heart—to devote time to what you need to bring into your life, or what someone else needs, to help make things happen. When I'm fearful, part of the fearfulness is sensing that the odds are overwhelmingly against me. I feel swept around like a tumbling leaf. Prayer gives me the courage to keep on.

Prayer is also a way of renewing. It's a time to reconnect to what matters, not just to beseech, *Oh, help me, please!* My friend Kelley calls it doing her gratitudes. I take moments in ceremony to feel what I'm grateful for. When I pray, I can reflect on what's precious to me, and when I think about that, I get more and more fed: I have a home in the beautiful wilderness. I have a vision that compels me. I teach Yoga and love doing it. How great is that? I am loved and I love; since I went through a good part of my life without that, I know how precious that is. Praying means taking the time to actually feel that sense of gratitude. Thinking is a lovely sport, but just thinking without feeling isn't enough to make it real.

I also pray for others. Just because I'm in the middle of my own storm doesn't mean I can't feel for others, and helping others renews me. In order to pray for someone else's healing, I must first tap in to these vast pools of energy inside me, and that's exhilarating; I feel better for it.

As a Medicine Person, people often request of me, "Send me some light. I need it."

I recently went into ceremony for a friend who'd just had abdominal surgery and was in terrible pain. I focused on draining her pain, praying that her scar tissue would be minimal, that my beloved friend's suffering would ease and she'd be surrounded by those who love her. And I didn't even realize that I needed to feel that loving connection with her as much as I needed to help her. In doing so, I also received tremendous healing.

People often ask me who I pray to, and the answer is to the spiritual beings I call the Sacred Ones, the beloved dead, yours and mine. I don't expect these entities to come in and fix the problem. I'm asking them for energy, time, and space. You may have a different name in mind: God, the Silence, the Spirit that Moves Through All Things. Find out what works for you and do it.

When I first began praying, my own prejudices came up in my face. For years I'd clung to the belief that there was no God, or if there was, God wouldn't be interested in me. I decided to experiment. What would happen if I prayed anyway, even if I had no faith? Even if prayer wouldn't help me, maybe it would help others, so it was worth doing. There are things larger than our beliefs. Forces in the universe work beyond our faith and knowledge. When you interact with them, life is much more fascinating.

Belief has power, but it is not all-powerful. I thank everything that is sacred because my beliefs have been pretty crappy. I can breathe in a faithless way and still get something out of it. If you have no reason to have faith, know that change is possible. I had faith in nothing, and now I have faith in many things. It's a new truth for me. I now have faith that I can make it through a hardship because I've done it so many times. My faith is built from my own experience of what works.

At first, when learning prayer, I found I couldn't pray to some white-haired, bearded angry guy in the sky; I had no interest in asking that kind of entity for anything. Someone tried to teach me the Zen tradition of bowing, but it wasn't for me. I'm not interested in any entity, person, or supernatural that needs me to bow or become smaller. I didn't need to be less for anybody.

I pray for what I want to have in my life. Some people say, "God will imagine it much better than you can," but I know that the Sacred Ones have a strange sense of humor, so I've learned to be specific. If I ask for a beloved, for example, I've figured out that I better pray that I'll be able to recognize that person, and that the person can't be dead. Once I prayed for a lover and got everything I asked for in a bird. I went back to the drawing board and my pipe: *Yes, that was a very pretty bird, but it has to be a mammal.* Then I got a cat. Back again. This time, I got a woman. *No, no, no, I need a man.* This was the way the Sacred Ones taught me to be specific about what I want but to leave an opening so it can be greater than I imagine. When I pray for something specific, I can track whether it actually happens. However, when I pray for something grandiose and vague—peace in the world, say—I can't track that.

Ask for what you want rather than what you *don't* want. Instead of saying, "I don't want to be controlled by my abuse anymore," say, "I want to walk free of my abuse," or, "Help me to free my life from my abuse." If you're always praying, *Release this, release that,* don't be surprised if you suddenly develop pervasive diarrhea!

I personally don't think it's wrong to ask for prosperity in your life. I want to be free of the burden of debts, but I see prosperity first and foremost as emotional, mental, physical, and spiritual health; that's real wealth. Pray to develop the tools and skills to get that if you don't have it. If you're financially stuck, pray to learn how to get financially healthy. If you're stuck around money, ask for what you need to learn to move those clogs out of your life. However, money needs to be able to stop somewhere in your life, so ask for balance so it doesn't flow right out.

Sometimes you can ask for specific tools, or you can simply say, "I want to let go. Make it happen." It's our job to grow and evolve, but we have to be active in that process. To sit back and wait like a baby for everything to be brought to us is immature and lazy.

I'm enchanted by the story of the woman who called herself Peace Pilgrim. Between 1953 and 1981, she walked more than 25,000 miles around the country to inspire others toward peace. To her, every step was prayer. I love that concept. Care enough about your prayers and intent to take some action.

The artifacts used in ceremony help because they focus people's attention, especially mine when I pray with my pipe. Following the Native American tradition of Calling in the Four Directions for protection takes time because I'll wait for something inside or outside to tell me what to say next. Sometimes I can't tell the difference. Is it my own heart or Spirit, or is it the Sacred Ones? I don't always know. While ceremony is helpful, sometimes you just don't have time. If life is urgent or I'm exhausted, I may do prayers in the shower; that's all the juice I have. I have learned to honor that.

Pray in whatever way feels authentic to you. Ultimately prayer can help you discover the answer to two important questions: *How can I walk through this situation in a way that I can be proud of? Even if my life is chaos, how can I still connect with that which is sacred?*

PHYSICAL FOCUS:
YOGA AND INTUITION

Our Yoga practice can provide a private, safe arena in which we can begin developing and flexing our intuitive muscles. By listening to our internal signals, we begin to experiment and play with how to use these buried and suffocated parts of ourselves. For example, as you are moving more deeply into a Yoga pose, listen and feel for your first edge of resistance. When your body resists, it's saying, *Wait.* If you wait and breathe into that tugging place, there can be an opening like an internal flowering that upgrades and sweetens the quality of energy you have inside in that moment. If you just barge on past that signal, occupied with where you think you should be in the pose, you're shunning the voice of your body's intelligence and missing that sweetness! Treat yourself with the honor and respect that you have been craving and you deserve. Yes, you do deserve honor and respect! If I do, so do you!

Let's say you're deep in a pose, you feel some pain, and you get a flash of something. How do you know whether you're having a somatic response to an intuitive signal or whether the pain is simply your body's reaction to reaching its edge? Is there a painful story to excavate beneath the pain? Breathe, feel, and wait for more information. When you're beginning to intuit, you'll make a lot of mistakes at first; allow it. Mistakes are a necessary part of learning.

As best as you can, locate where you're feeling the sensation in your body. Inhale deeply, reaching for or into the painful area; feel it all the way through inhale and exhale. Keep feeling through the area; shifting mental gears, changing thinking to feeling. Then give it space by expanding the area with your breath. Breathing has a physiological effect; the fresh oxygen stimulates the blood supply, the body's natural way of healing. It breaks up the stagnation; things can't heal in a stagnant pond. Pain is often trapped energy, so as the block releases, it might become more painful at first; most of us go a little numb around hurt, especially chronic pain, because that's the only way we know how to cope. But as you breathe deeply, the numbness and pain recede.

Get curious about tracking the quality of different sensations you might feel instead of freaking out because any sensation equals pain—*Oh my god, I'm feeling my back!* Just feel what you feel. Heat, cold, itchiness? Feel every little quiver. It's all information. You might feel a flickering of fearfulness. Part of what's creating painful blockages are the emotions we have about them—sad, scary thoughts about what that pain means for us. *I'm trapped. I can't hold myself up. I'll always feel this way.* Breathe that away; reclaim what you once disowned in order to survive.

Iris had a lot of pain, tightness, and sometimes numbness in her upper back. I taught her Shoulder Shrugs in Warrior II (see page 64) and got her breathing into the area. Slowly, as Iris breathed into her upper back, she began to get flashes of a deeper emotional pain. Soon she connected the pain in her back with a difficult work situation about which she felt helpless. A coworker wanted her job, and Iris felt that colleague was stabbing her in the back. Her body's response was a literal interpretation of that feeling. More feelings came up for Iris—she was sad and freaked out that someone hated her for how good she was at her job, but the more she spoke this deeper truth, the more the muscle tissue began to soften and become even more responsive. I asked, "What's it feel like in there?" "It's a little sore, but it doesn't feel like I'm carrying this big backpack anymore," Iris told me. Listening more deeply to her body helped her excavate a story that gave voice to her pain and began to resolve it.

All of the poses are teachers for learning to listen within; follow your Ujjayi breath inward. Feeling more and more how the breath and energy move inside you is part of developing the skill of learning to listen to and feel your intuition.

LYING OVER A ROLL

If you don't get all that indigestible, nonnutritive garbage out of the way, you can't listen to what your body is trying to tell you. Lying over a Roll helps you literally move that crap out of the way while bringing a tremendous amount of vitality to your belly so your gut feelings are literally clearer. Gut feelings are part of intuitive communication. When someone walks into the room and your stomach drops, there's a reason for that; that's your intuition talking.

Place the roll at your navel, between the pubic bone and your ribs. Relax into that intensity in your core—it helps break up what's blocking energy in there. It also moves out back pain, which can be very distract-ing—and when you're distracted, you're not a good listener.

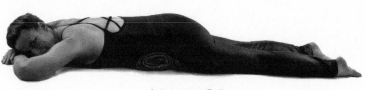

Lying over a Roll

The gift of intuition comes to those who practice with patience. This is why so many more Silver Hairs are intuitive. Recently, Heyoka and I were laughing about the fact that he is the oldest Sun Dancer in his group of Crow Dancers. He's seventy now. We've become the elders we once watched and learned from.

Friend do it this way—that is,
whatever you do in life,
do the very best you can
with both your heart and mind.
And if you do it that way,
the Power of the Universe
will come to your assistance,
if your heart and mind are in Unity.
When one sits in the Hoop of the People,
one must be responsible because
All of Creation is related.
And the hurt of one is the hurt of all.
And the honor of one is the honor of all.
And whatever we do affects everything in the universe.
If you do it that way—that is, if you truly join your heart and mind
as One—whatever you ask for,
that's the Way It's Going to Be.

From the teachings of White Buffalo Calf Woman

8

EMBODYING SPIRIT:
ROMANCING THE SOUL

I WAS SITTING inside the sweat lodge on Heyoka's property in Washington. The lodge was a pretty upside-down willow basket connected by bailing wire covered with sacred red ties at the joints. That day it was just a bare frame; we only covered it with blankets when we were doing a sweat. Nestled into a secret hollow in the hill, it offered me a view of the house, and out east, down the hill was the big wide Columbia River. It was fairly calm that day, although I'd seen the wind whip up big waves at other times. To the west was the willow where Heyoka and I did our Sun Dances to talk to the Sacred Ones for guidance during the summer. To the south was the stream, which was almost always talking; Heyoka and I liked to go out there and eat lunch amid the flowers and the miniature lily pads of miner's lettuce, which tasted sweet and bitter and green with so much life that bursts in your mouth. To the north was Heyoka's round-domed house.

I'd gone inside the lodge to pray, to ask for connection for my solitary soul. There was a healing that was happening on the rez. The tribe members had endured tremendous loss and defeat at the hands of white people. The white people had earned a reputation as thieves, liars, and destroyers. It was a slow and careful walk for me through that minefield of fear and hate in order to learn and carry the medicine traditions. Like the Native Americans, I knew what it was to be lied to, stolen from, and destroyed. I used this as a doorway to walk into medicine.

Now, in winter, snow fell everywhere, flakes fluttering down between the willow poles and landing on me where I sat, knees pulled up tight to my chest. As I huddled there in the cold, trying to calm my mind, the thunder and lightning began.

Heyoka told me later that thunder and lightning and snow don't mix—yet I've had this happen many times for me. As I sat there listening, it was as though I could hear something beyond the thunder. There were no actual words, but something was definitely communicating with me. I listened intently. First rumbling, then little murmurs. It would stop, then start up again. Sometimes I had to strain to hear it. It was obviously talking to me, in the same way that when a horse blows at you, it's talking to you, but what it's saying gets lost in translation. It was up to me to stretch and hear what the thunder was telling me. The sound drummed right down into my bone marrow—not because it was loud and deafening, but because it was so resonant. It was bringing something dead inside of me back to life.

The Thunder Kachina, or Spirits, were talking to me! I had the sense that it was affectionate contact—something really big having communication with really small me. The message was clear: I mattered. My growly, bitchy self meant something to the Sacred Ones. This broke my heart open.

That was an actual experience of that which moves in all things, what the Native Americans call *Wakan Skan,* or Sacred Mystery—a concept of Spirit I understand down to my bones. My beliefs grow from my experience. I have communion and relationship with the Sacred Ones.

My experience in the lodge was proof of a deep connection to this larger Spirit. It shook the old delusional beliefs about my worthlessness right out of me and into the ground. I could no longer deny the truth of that which moves in all things also flowing through me.

It felt as if I was being drawn to Spirit inch by slow inch. Perhaps that was the only way this stubborn self would accept it. I'd had my vision of Mending the Rainbow Hoop of the People. I'd had this experience of that which moves in all things. And then something else happened that gave me the momentum I needed to keep moving toward my mission.

It was the dead of winter. I woke up from a guilt-filled dream about abandoning my horse all those years ago when I was in the grip of drinking and drugging—Chelsey, my white magic horse with the blue eyes, my beauty who looked like a unicorn who'd lost her horn. I'd sold her to a reputable school, but I still felt so awful about giving up on this very gentle, kind being. I got up, still caught in the web of the terrible dream, pulled a jacket on over my naked body, thrust my bare feet into snow boots, and stumbled out to the outhouse. Slipping and sliding down the hill, I clumped inside the outhouse to pee. Looking out the open door down at the Columbia River, I could see something was down there. I couldn't quite tell what, but I felt some strange compulsion to find out. I ran straight down the mountain to the little cliff above the river where Heyoka and I had built a medicine wheel, a stone circle ten feet across, with a line of stones and precious objects we used for ceremony running from the center to each of the Four Directions—North, East, South, and West. Not quite understanding why, I ran around the medicine wheel sunwise three times. Then I looked down the cliff, and bathed in silver moonlight was a deer on the little sand patch between the cliff and the river.

We stared at each other for a while. It was a magic moment. At some point I sent a picture question to her: *Name?* I thought I was asking the deer her name, not connecting that in ceremony, I had been asking for my name as a Medicine Woman. The deer sent back a response so clearly, it was as though she'd spoken the words aloud: *Shy Ayla.* I told the deer in mental pictures, *Stay here. I'll be right back.* I went running back up the hill, slipping and sliding through the snow, and pawed through the makeshift kitchen until I found an apple and an English muffin. Then I went running back down, pausing once again to run around the medicine wheel three times. The deer was standing in the exact same spot. I held out the apple and the muffin—*Come, you can have them*—but she didn't approach to eat them. Then I saw what I hadn't seen before: her back leg had been almost shot off; it was hanging on by the skin. She was obviously suffering, close to death. I put down the apple and the English muffin close to her and told her, *Wait here,* again without words.

I went and got Heyoka; together we ran around the wheel three times. Suddenly it hit me: Deer is keeper of magic. I made the connection: Chelsey was my magic horse; now I was being visited by a Magic Keeper. She was here to remind me that it was time to pick up my own magic.

Heyoka lifted his rifle to his shoulder, shot the deer at point-blank range, and somehow missed. She jumped at the gun's report but stayed rooted to the spot. She must have been in unimaginable pain. I started crying. *It won't be long now,* I told her without words. It took three shots. On the third shot, she just folded up her legs and fell down as gracefully as a dancer. There was hardly any blood; she must have nearly bled out before. I walked over and petted her as the brightness in her eyes dimmed.

I dragged her back up that icy mountain. On the way she grew to the size of a full-blown elk. I felt like Sisyphus dragging the rock to infinity. We got a tarp, dragged her into the house, and butchered her. We took the heart and liver and left them as an offering for my eagles and crows in the feeding tree, which was down by the river right where she had been standing. She had old bullet wounds in her. Her body was so infected, it was filled with pus. Her death was an offering of her magic, not her flesh. We took it in bags to the dump, but sent the skin off to be tanned. I took her head and placed it on the crotch of a nearby tree by the stream, and asked the creepy crawlies to please clean this Medicine Person for me. When spring finally came, I went to that same tree, but there was no skull on it. Then I looked down at my feet and saw a partial skull with antlers and marveled at this transition: I had put her skull there as a gift; however, what I got in return was a partial skull with antlers. Today it sits in my own home in my medicine room in the East, in the little crow's nest, thirty feet above the ground. This powerful medicine gift is still working with me today.

Sometime after that, we visited Tom Yellowtail, an old Medicine Man in Montana. I asked him about the deer and the name, Shy Ayla. "What did it mean? Whose name was that?" Tom replied: "Well, she wasn't looking for a name, was she? Who was looking for a name?" I learned from some other folks that Shyayla was the Lakota name for the Cheyenne people. It means "Shield of Her People."

Yet again, my old script that I wasn't worthy had been shattered. I wasn't totally ready to walk free of the strictures of that old belief, but now it was like a shadow web, not a sturdy prison. That deer gave me her death, her skin, and my medicine name; what incredible gifts.

There was a change in the wind. A friend of mine named Madaline Blau had come up to the rez for a visit, and we'd done a healing on someone on New Year's Eve. It had been a bad night for this man; he'd mixed prescription drugs with alcohol. His blood pressure was about to blow through the roof. Miraculously, he improved after our healing. Suddenly, there was talk—not *Hey, these people saved this guy's life!* but *Oh no, this woman is a witch!* Then someone stuck a cow's skull on one of the trees on our land and set it on fire. A warning to everyone—*Stay away from the witch!* A warning to me: *Leave! We don't want your evil magic.* It was a time of great reckoning. I had begun to realize that what I most needed from Heyoka wasn't anything he could give. I'd learned so much being with him, and it had been an important and often sacred time for me, but it was time to go.

Much earlier, I'd started work on another piece of beading. I felt like when I finished that, I would be free to go. It would be my masterpiece—something I created for the express purpose of selling it to buy my own land. It is an incredibly ambitious design: an Appaloosa looking into the viewer's face. On this horse I beaded hoof prints, stripes, and a lightning bolt (for lightning medicine); I beaded a feather into her tail and an old-fashioned saddle on her back, with a crimson blanket, rifle, and a silver crow shield, to symbolize the Sweet Medicine of the crows I'd come to love on the rez. There is a thunderhead in the sky, a blanket of rain and lightning, a medicine wheel where ceremony is taking place. I beaded a bowl and a cloud of smoke transforming into a dragon coming out of the bowl. My medicine pipe lies next to the bowl. The outer edge of the frame is deerskin, to honor deer medicine. I called this piece "Ceremony of Calling in the Dream."

The beads are nearly microscopic; this tiny beadwork masterpiece took me more than a year to complete, but if it could buy me the freedom of my own land, it was worth the sacrifice. As I worked the final beads into place, it felt like another sign: *My time here is finished.* (As it turned out, I didn't have to sell the piece after all. I found out that I could keep the beauty I created and still have what I wanted.) Today, my bead masterpiece hangs in my sunrise dome-home.

I'd run from Rosalyn to the rez. My time there had given me so many gifts: the teachings of Medicine People, the beginnings of connection to Spirit. I took a final walk over to the trees where my beloved crows had brought me regular Sweet Medicine reports. Over the years I'd come to love my relationship with the four-foots and my winged friends; in many ways our communication had been deeper than what I'd had with most of the two-foots on the rez. Then it was time to leave. I tossed what little I owned into my truck and barreled on out of there.

As I drove back toward California, I continued to reflect on the vision I'd had of myself back on the rez. How could I send rainbow hoops of healing around the world? By the time I got back to Santa Monica, I knew the answer. It was time to open something of my very own: Forrest Yoga Circle. Putting my name on my studio was a declaration that I was ready to step more fully into my mission. I didn't want my Yoga studio to be just about pretty poses. I wanted to help people heal at a more profound level, to help them seek a deep spiritual connection and find more adventure. I felt that using Yoga to connect, interact, and romance with your Spirit was as sexy as you could get.

The studio had only been open a few weeks when I got my first flash on how I might begin to enact my vision of Mending the Hoop of the People. A message came to me during pipe ceremony: *Heal the holes in the ozone.*

When I had been living with Heyoka, I'd once gone into ceremony for four days at the request of a long-distance friend whose cervix was effacing prematurely; she was struggling to hold on to her baby. As I sat with my pipe, a spider crawled toward me. After I got over my city girl reaction—*Ugh, a spider! Kill it!*—I asked myself, *Is this a medicine sign? What does it mean?* I realized: oh, a weaver, baskets, uterus. That's what I needed to do: weave a supportive energetic basket around my friend's uterus. Weaving is traditionally women's work. I energetically laid my friend down on the floor and wove and wove. A few hours later she called me: "What did you do? I'm walking around. I'm not bleeding." She and the baby were absolutely fine until she went into labor. Then she had to have a C-section because she couldn't dilate enough—guess I wove that cervix too tight! I swear, that little baby boy—now a gorgeous and sulky young man—has been angry at me his whole life!

Could I heal the ozone layer by weaving it closed? I'd learned on the reservation how to focus *for* something. I explained to my students that we needed to align with something necessary and greater than ourselves, like healing the ozone layer of our atmosphere. I decided we would do an Ozone Healing Meditation every Friday night in Santa Monica. (The strangeness of a group gathering to heal the ozone layer attracted a physicist, who later became my second husband.) It was amazing; the students were really into it, and every week more people showed up! Our energetic work was like dealing with the proud flesh of horses all over again—first we had to clean out the jagged, gunky perimeters of the ozone holes so they could heal and bond. Then we'd energetically weave over the holes.

I would set the intent—"We're going to focus more on cleanup"— and then fifteen minutes before the end of the meditation, I'd announce, "Finishing up now." Then I'd ask my students: "What did you see? What did you do?" Something powerful and profound was happening; we all felt it—somehow we were aligning with what was needed on a planetary level. One guy told me, "I saw a million million spiders weaving"—I'd never told him about the spider's presence as I healed my friend's cervix. The students' visions started to become congruent. After a few months, I learned that the Earth Summit in Rio de Janeiro was taking place—a radical new development. While we were doing our meditation, these high-powered people were brainstorming at a conference. What good medicine!

I began acting on messages I received through those meditations. One day I drove by a huge billboard with a picture of a little girl pointing a gun out to the viewer (me) with the words *Stop the Violence*. I saw the violence that we apply to ourselves and to each other and how it continues to add to the heat of our planet and create problems like the holes in the ozone. We needed to stop the violence we do to ourselves and to each other. I began talking to my students about the importance of stopping self-mutilating talk, about honoring our bodies and our life experiences. The more I spoke from the heart, the more I felt I was honoring my name as Shield of Her People and doing my part to Mend the

Hoop of the People. I was at last beginning to embody and heed the call of my own Spirit. The more I honored it, the more brightly my Spirit burned within me.

After a whole year of doing these weekly Ozone Healing Meditations, I received another message: *Don't close the holes completely.* Those holes were there for a reason; they were chimneys for the heat to pass through, and we needed them until we could control our emissions. I told the group the message I'd received, and we stopped, just like that. I have no idea what it did, but I knew it was a necessary step, and I certainly received many gifts from it. One day maybe I'll learn why!

PUTTING OUT THE CALL TO SPIRIT

Spirit is the sacred essence within each person. We're born with it, but it doesn't necessarily stay with us; it can be shocked out of our bodies. I've seen Spirits gone quiescent, there but hiding. I've seen Spirits leave. Some Spirits come and go. I'd been hunting something very elusive for seventeen years—my own Spirit. It had taken me a long time to find it— my authentic self, which had been smothered under all those layers of shame, guilt, fear, and pain. I had to disrupt those layers before there was any room inside of me for my Spirit to live. Life on the reservation, and my choice to take action on my life's mission, had given me the chance to call my Spirit home. When I found it, I was determined to keep my Spirit nourished and delighted so it would stay—that took me a while. Once I discovered that first conscious pathway of reconnecting to Spirit, I didn't want to walk anywhere else. Yet it's still daunting to realize I can lose touch with my precious essence again if I don't stay mindful.

I want to teach you how to put out a call to your Spirit and keep it delighted so it will stay. Put into play the following exercises to romance your soul. Your Spirit needs to be delighted. Together we will walk in Beauty. Exploring and learning how to live in Beauty is a holistic view of the world that acknowledges the need to accept both the good and the bad in everything; part of connecting with Spirit is to walk in Beauty. I'll also show you how to clean out your spiritual smog. If you want your Spirit to come home to stay, you'll need to keep alert for depressing, smog-bearing thought emissions that could drive it out.

In the "Physical Focus" section of the chapter, I'll help you get a more visceral feel for what living with Spirit feels like by first practicing its opposite—what I call endarkenment. I'll offer instructions on how to use breath as an invitation to Spirit. Then I'll review the Yoga poses that are especially beneficial in opening the body to the sparkling energy that delights the Spirit.

SPIRITUAL FOCUS:
EXERCISES TO ROMANCE THE SOUL

You don't have to be on the mountaintop to connect to Spirit. I teach people how to find Spirit on the mat, but you could just as easily connect to it at home, on the way to work, at the store. Wherever you are, start by reflecting on why connecting to your Spirit would be meaningful for you. What part of you wouldn't benefit if you were connected to Spirit? Why wouldn't you want that blessing in your life? How about the part of you that is wedded to the lies that keep you small and shutdown and controlled? I challenge you to risk going through your fears and explore connecting your Spirit into your body, living and practicing embodying Spirit. When you can feel your Spirit is intact, even the ordinary moments of your life become extraordinary. When you're embodying Spirit, you can look at another person and your eyes will rest there in wonder and awe.

Do you believe that you don't have enough time to call in Spirit? I spend around two hundred fifty days on the road every year. I have learned I can put out a call to Spirit even when I'm standing in a security line at the airport.

Whether it's your connection to your Spirit that has been broken or your Spirit itself has been shattered, there are ways to bring it home to your body and heal it. To walk the path of your Spirit, staying mindful begins the journey. It's about the quality of attention. When does this mindfulness become automatic? Never. To dwell in Spirit, stay out of automatic mode. Evolving is conscious, not robotic. You walk, you fall. Falling is just part of the journey, so stop making such a damn drama about it and just get up.

PUTTING OUT A CALL TO SPIRIT

If you honestly don't feel Spirit, put out a call to it and leave a psychic voicemail. Ask whatever power you believe in, or wish you could believe in, to help you connect. I know; it feels risky to actually pray or ask for what you want. Risk doing it anyway.

Spirit rides on breath and is fed by the inhale and exhale. With breath you can invite your Spirit back in. To entice my Spirit, I had to allow myself to breathe so I could feel an incredibly effervescent, *alive* sparkle spreading through my body; my breath was the sweetest ambrosia. At the same time I felt this scintillating sparkle, I was overcome by a bittersweet feeling that made me cry out of control. In connecting to my Spirit, I had to feel the pain of how long I'd been disconnected, and that pain was excruciating. I had to feel through the grieving of it. I kept shutting down.

Then I had to suffer my way through a lot of stupid thoughts: *Now that I'm connected to my Spirit, x, y, and z are going to happen.* Not true, they didn't. I also had to get beyond the belief, *Now that I've found Spirit, I'll never lose that connection.* I was wrong. I did. I had to keep breathing and feeling deeper and deeper into those emotions—the ecstatic sweetness and euphoria, including the terror of losing it and the hesitance to feel the ecstasy because of the fear of losing it—experiencing wave after unbearable wave. All my conditions and reasons for staying numb had to be blown out until I could go deeper through the emotions and establish the reconnection.

Set your intent to call in Spirit and then explore breathing in a way that connects you to Spirit. Sit up straight and take deep, strong breaths with the intent to blow out the internal smog and cobwebs. Bring in fresh energy. Keeping your eyes closed, breathe in a way that literally brightens you up internally; you may even see a brightness or lightening behind your eyelids. Start acknowledging that you're doing something good for yourself. This acknowledgment starts to coax your Spirit back into your body. You may sense a subtle or obvious change in your energy. Feel for the visceral signs that your Spirit is coming forth. Sometimes you'll experience a bittersweet, sorrowful crying, as though your heart were being washed with tears. It is. Let it come. Usually my students show their connection to their Spirit with actual tears as soon as they let go of some of their shields. They actually glow.

If you've been separated from your Spirit for a long time—or have never felt it before—when you recognize it coming forth, you may paradoxically feel, as I did, a great sadness because the painfulness of that separation becomes even more obvious and the sweetness of finally coming home and connecting to your Spirit is so heartfilling! Cherish that feeling.

When you feel the connection to Spirit, ask: *What can I do for you today?* I have learned that my Spirit needs breath, attention, challenge, adventure, beauty, and love. Discovering what I need to heal myself or another who is bereft also feeds my Spirit. Just because you have a conscious mind doesn't mean that you know what your Spirit needs. Don't assume you know. This is part of romancing your soul. Ask your beloved Spirit and learn. Do a few Yoga poses, working to get your breath conscious. Feel for spreading the energy through your fingertips. Instead of feeling how far can you go in the pose or how long can you stay in it, how long can you feel your Spirit exploring the physical pose? Build a repertoire of what feeds your Spirit and work up to making that your daily practice.

If you can't feel any connection to your Spirit, don't give up. Do this: breathe deeply into your heart. Your faith isn't important in this moment; you just need to connect to your heart. It's there keeping you alive, whether you believe it or not. Put your hand on your heart, send warmth to it, and ask: *What can I do for you today?* Keep breathing into your heart until you get a response. You might not be able to discern an answer; that happens. Just allow for that and experiment, do something for your heart anyway. There's no need to go huge by asking something like *What does my heart want to do for my life's dream?* Instead, take a small, manageable step—take three breaths into your heart. Want to go bigger? Then take a walk around the block and continue breathing into your heart. That's a really good start. Take baby steps every day. As your heart gets nourished and becomes responsive, put out a heartfelt call, using your heart's new strength to help guide Spirit home.

WALKING WITH BEAUTY

Another way to connect with Spirit is to walk with Beauty. This way, you respond to adversity not from fear, but from an honest, intelligent place. You can look at adversity as merely a series of problems, or you can see it as a test that makes you a great problem solver. Seeing life this way doesn't mean surrendering. It means you recognize the truth of what is. You can't stop a meteor from shooting across the sky, but you can revel in its mystery and Beauty. You can't stop a flash flood—but you can learn to get out of the canyon if you don't want to become good food for the crows.

Recall that Beauty with a capital *B* refers to a Native American perception of the world, one that embraces balance, harmony, and the essential correctness of the bad informing the good and vice versa. It's about seeing the exquisiteness of the whole cycle—birth, life, death. Beauty isn't only out there, waiting for us to notice it; it exists with or without us. It's within us and informs how we walk in the world. We create Beauty and put it out into the multiverse. Walking with Beauty means accepting that the (perceived) bad is part of everything. If someone you love gets fatal cancer, viewed from a Beauty way, perhaps that's how the person is doing the death dance. Tragedy, sadness: everything is part of Beauty.

When you shift your perception of life from victim mode—*Everything bad happens to me*—or judging mode—*This is great, this sucks*—and shift to a curiosity and a desire to more fully discern the truth, then you are walking with Beauty. You're living more authentically from a place of Spirit.

Look at your world. How marvelous a tree is! Notice the bark pattern, the new leaves, the bizarre roots pushing through the sidewalk, instead of focusing on them as a nuisance that you stumbled over. Did it take stumbling over them to see them? Look at the sky, the clouds, the stars; revel in them. Look at this fabulous, mysterious place we live in. Why not touch the Sacred and the Great Mystery on the way to pick up your coffee? You can make life richer moment by moment. You don't need to go to a Yoga retreat to have those experiences. Within the ordinary is the extraordinary.

Make walking with Beauty a fun game. Take time to pet the cat and actually feel her silky fur and notice her happy response; that's a Beauty moment. Instead of thinking about your stressful financial situation, take a moment, take a breath, connect to your cat. Keep breathing and then find one step that you can take that will be helpful to your stressful financial situation. When your kids are begging for something from you, instead of responding with that tired "Yes, honey, what do you want?" can you take that moment and make it a real interaction so you and your child have something of worth?

Looking at Beauty helps connect you to something beyond your problems. Beauty Moments aren't only for moments of stress; they're necessary for a healthy Spirit—a Spirit that wants to be fed, played with, given choices. Make connecting to them part of your daily diet for the Spirit.

It can be harder to see Beauty within our relationships. We can become so caught up in the energetic charge of our resentment toward others—how they're not meeting our needs, all the stuff they're not doing for us—that we lose sight of who they really are. Focus instead on what you love in them. I'm not saying, "Shut up and quit complaining." Just don't dig into that same old trench of resentment and dissatisfaction—if you dig in, so do they! When you challenge yourself to see the whole person in your boss, employee, or mate, you'll have a richer experience.

My manager and I had fallen into a dynamic of sharing only problems. My life on the road is incredibly hectic, and she is the air traffic controller who has to manage thousands of details. Our conversations had fallen into a rut about fixing whatever was wrong, usually on a tight schedule. I was slow to realize that she wasn't there to witness and drink from the Beauty of the Yoga ceremonies that nourished me and my students, so she was getting only a one-sided picture of my life and the job. We'd both become disheartened. So we decided to start and end our business meetings with a Beauty Report. That smoothed the dissonance between us.

CLEARING OUT YOUR SPIRITUAL SMOG

If you want your Spirit to come home, stop indulging the behavior that drives it away. You know, this repulsive behavior in which you think your most depressing, spiritual-smog-bearing thoughts. What you do internally keeps your Spirit or drives it out. You might have created a mess that you need to clean up, but as long as you can feel the sacredness of your Spirit, you can fill yourself with its sparkliness; then you won't need to indulge in those poisonous thoughts that drive Spirit out.

I once had a vision of myself walking down the street, arguing in my head with various people. I was doing my usual internal target practice, taking aim at all the people I was angry at. *Pow. Pow. Pow.* Suddenly my perspective switched into an overview. It was as though I were an eagle, looking down on this Ana person and seeing who she really was. I saw this incredible psychic shit pouring out of me, my own personal filthy smog. Here I was, filled with this magnificent vision of Mending the Hoop of the People, and yet this toxic nonsense was what I was actually giving to the world! That was a powerful medicine experience. I could no longer be oblivious to the effect I was truly having in the world, the consequences of my actions *right now,* in every moment.

It's not enough to put out a call to your Spirit. Also become aware when you give in to smoggy, negative thinking; set your intention to radiate brightness instead.

CREATING AND LIVING THE ETHICS OF YOUR SPIRIT

Why have you lived the way you have to this point? It's because you've been guided by a personal code of ethics—what I define as the rules, guidelines, values, and goals, both conscious and unconscious, which shape your behaviors. When you begin to walk the path of your Spirit, choose to examine those ethics and see if they're leading you toward your more authentic self—the key to unlocking Spirit—or miring you in self-sabotaging behaviors that block you from Spirit.

Whatever we choose not to examine, we carry with us or perpetuate unconsciously. This is especially true for our ethics. We learn these primarily from our parents or caretakers, teachers, religious leaders, and friends. Unfortunately, what we probably learned from them sounds something like *Do as I say, not as I do.* We think of the internal tape inside our head as the unimpeachable voice of our ethical coach, but in fact it's usually quite insane and vicious. The parent says, "Strive more. Strive more," and the babe hears, "You're not enough. You're not enough." The priest or rabbi tells us, "You must do this or you're a bad person." The teacher tells us, "You flunked; you're stupid." Our friends tell us, "Do this or you're not cool." Those disempowering voices get hardwired into our brains and rule our lives unless we challenge them. When we move from unconscious obedience to those rules, we can create new ethics that are rewarding and thrilling to live by.

The easiest way to begin developing your own ethics is to explore how you like to be treated. Do you have rules for this that are different from how you treat others? Realize too that others may not want to be treated as you like being treated. Can you treat someone as they'd like to be treated if it doesn't compromise you in any way?

The way you live your ethics also reflects your relationship to the truth. Often your ethics will reveal whether you have been wounded in your life and will give clues as to how these wounds are healing. If the truth has been used to hurt you, you may believe that being truthful isn't always worthwhile.

Your ethics will change as you consciously work on them and gather more life experience. I divide ethics into four categories:

Goal Ethics: These define who you want to grow into and what guidelines will help you develop into that person.

Action Ethics: These are the actions that will help you become who you want to grow into. Action Ethics are what you *do* and *live now.* For example, if one of your Goal Ethics is to become a published novelist and to accomplish this, you need to create an original plot and write a two-hundred-fifty-page manuscript and shop it around to literary agents, your Action Ethic would be to create a writing schedule that you can honestly follow with appropriate deadlines for an outline, sample chapters, and the like.

Taproot Ethics: These are the actions you're already taking to move toward your goals. For example, you may already be researching literary agencies, taking notes for plot points, dreaming up characters, creating a sacred time for daily writing, and so on. Identifying the Taproot Ethics by which you're already living honors the work you've done. It also keeps you from perpetuating a state of neediness and self-pity.

Entrapment Ethics: These are the so-called rules that sabotage your attempts to move forward, the false beliefs that keep you stuck. Perhaps you believe that only people with literary connections get published; you don't have a following, so no one will want to publish you; or you didn't get a fancy education, so who do you think you are trying to write a book? These beliefs hold you back from attaining your goals.

To find out what your ethics are, get out a pen and paper and answer these questions. What are your ethics regarding: Sex? Relationships? Power? Spirituality? Responsibility to self?

Next, ask yourself, *Where did these ethics come from? Parents, school, religion, friends?* If you borrowed or developed them based on the beliefs of others, was it a conscious decision? Next to each category of ethics, write down its origin. Now check yourself: Are these ethics really true for you? Have they brought you closer to your goals or taken you farther from them? Does your ethical code support you in becoming your wiser self? Do your ethics take into account your needs as well as healing, learning, growing, and nourishing your Spirit? Do they excite you? Do they make you proud? If not, redesign them!

Look back at the journaling you did for the Death Meditation in chapter four. What did you list as your priorities? How do your ethics support those?

Do your ethics support what's most meaningful to you? If not, rewrite them! What are your Goal Ethics now—who do you want to become? What Action Ethics do you need to take to walk more authentically on that path? What Taproot Ethics are already in place to support that? What Entrapment Ethics will you need to let go of to create your life as your personal masterpiece?

Test this new code of ethics. Does it work for you right now? Find out by living it. Make your ethics a living document that supports becoming your wiser self. When I created my own code of ethics, it required a lot of editing and rewriting and testing. The more I live by my ethics, the more easily I walk embodying Spirit. Here are some of my most meaningful ethics:

- Treat students with respect and honor for their unique walk and struggle.

- Use teaching to exercise my capacity to be loving and a Truth Speaker with grace.

- Speak, hear, see, touch, smell, feel, and walk truth, and teach others to do the same.

- Acknowledge when I have acted outside of integrity and correct the situation.

- Align my actions with my life vision, i.e., Does this action contribute to or take away from Mending the Hoop of the People?

- Exercise compassion for myself, for what I have not yet learned.

- Stay alert for my addictive behaviors sliding into action.

- Use this question to judge the correctness of my actions: Does this brighten or dim my Spirit?

- Nurture pleasure as a *Sadhana* (spiritual exercise) and relish evolving.

- Make time enough for love.

THE FUTURE/WISER SELF MEDITATION

I know from experience that it can be challenging to walk in Spirit. You might spend a lot of time fine-tuning your ethics, yet you will still stumble. You might find yourself questioning which direction will guide you in walking the path of your Spirit. When this happens, you will benefit enormously from the wisdom of an elder who's already walked that path.

Let me offer you a meditation/journaling process for connecting with your wiser self, inspired by Gloria Steinem, in which you create an arena to meet your older, wiser, more evolved self. This version of yourself knows the answers to the questions you have today, has lived through the struggles in the present, and has gained wisdom and perspective from them. This is the best person to guide you on your life path. This exercise can give you a blueprint for walking into the person you most yearn to be.

You need a quiet forty-five minutes or so and a place where you won't be disturbed. Let's do it now! Grab your notebook and write *Future/*

Wiser Self at the top of a fresh page—I have great hope that your future self will be wiser. Don't you? As I lead you through this meditation, take notes, answering the questions I pose.

Take some deep, spacious breaths. I want you to connect to a place. You may already know this place, you may have been there, or it may be a place that comes into being in your mind's eye. It is a place of great beauty that feels like the home to your soul. Everywhere you look, the beauty feeds you.

Now look around. There is a road, a path through this place of great beauty. Start walking down that path. Feel the earth beneath your feet. What does the air feel like? What scents are in the air? Are there flowers? Do you smell grass, ocean, trees? Inhale the smell of the sun-toasted rocks. Let all of your senses drink in from your sanctuary. Know that this is your life path that you are walking on.

Look ahead on your path. There is someone a little way ahead of you. This is your future self. It might be you from six months in the future or fifteen years. This future self has already walked through the challenges you are in right now. Your future self is a little more evolved, perhaps more at peace. Whatever it is you really want to grow into—there that person is, already growing into it. Your future self will be your guide here. Nobody knows you better than that future, wiser self.

Walk next to this person. Match strides with your future self. How do you feel about this person? Are you proud to be there with your wiser self? Ask any questions that you have; your future self has the answers. What do you need to know? Ask about your deeper troubling problems. Stay wide open for the response.

Match breath for breath with your future self. Then let the essence of your Spirit slide into the body of your future self so that you are actually walking *in* the body of the future you. What does that feel like? Smell this beautiful place as you walk. What's the difference in your senses? Now feel into the parts of your body where your past self has problems, for example, a back injury. Check it out in the body of your future self. Is that area still a problem?

Do you like your future self? What do self-respect and self-esteem feel like? How does your wiser self feel about your body and your problems? Is your future self still ruled by the beliefs of *I can't* or *I have to be perfect*? Is your future self still dealing with the challenges, blind spots, and weaknesses of your past self? Is there compassion for that past self? Is there contempt?

In your wisdom, don't you want to help your past self? Feel that truth inside. Tell your past self the keys to moving through life's challenges. Connecting even more deeply with the body of your wiser self, ask: *What unique gifts do I have to offer in this world? A generous heart? A curious mind? What do I have to offer to Mend the Hoop of the People?* Listen for the response.

Slide back into your present self, still walking beside your future self. Ask your wiser self what important things you must understand or do to become this person you most yearn to be. Ask your future self what you need to do to reconnect whenever you want to take counsel of that person's wisdom.

Look deeply into those eyes that understand you so completely. Is there anything else either of you wants to ask or say at this time?

Absorb the Beauty and the great mystery of your wiser self. Look around at your sanctuary, this exquisite place that is home for you. Stay connected to that Beauty. Come back with your awareness, to where you're sitting. Stay lightly connected to your wiser self and this beautiful place.

The Meditation with Your Future, Wiser Self will guide you in walking the path of your Spirit. Reflect on it often. Pledge to do what is necessary to become this person you most yearn to be, and write down your pledge. Now, in addition to your code of ethics, you have another good way to measure your actions: does whatever you're doing bring you closer to your future self, or does it take you down your old path?

What can you do today and tomorrow that will walk you on the path to your future, wiser self? What ethics do you need to have in place to become that person? Invite all the information you just learned to live in your body. Give this information a home in your cell tissue; let it soak in. Bring that sparkly energy in! Now have a blast with being the person you most want to be. Why wait? Do it now.

PHYSICAL FOCUS:
FROM ENDARKENMENT TO LIGHTENING

My students struggle when they first reach for and consciously connect with their Spirit; they're not sure if what they're feeling is authentic. Riding the breath is the easiest way to meet your Spirit. Deep breathing while in Yoga poses will help you tap in to the exhilarating energy of your Spirit. Choose poses that aren't too challenging so you won't get tangled in doing the pose. Frequently when we struggle, we lose our ability to feel our Spirit. It's like trying to relax in the midst of a fight. Choose a pose and be struggle-free in it, staying focused on coaching your Spirit to respond to the pose.

Abs with a Roll and Frog Lifting Through (see pages 59–60) are great poses to help brighten from your core and create internal connection and vitality. I encourage you to breathe in a way that releases any ongoing clamping down, holding, or habitual tension in the body. Cross-Legged Side Bend (see page 61) and Chest Opener on the Wall (see pages 92–93) are also very powerful poses to invite your Spirit in. But just doing the poses isn't going to help; you have to do the poses while coaching the Spirit in.

While in these poses, feel for the visceral signs that your Spirit is participating. If you've been separated from your Spirit for a long time, you may feel both the incredible sweetness of finally coming home and connecting to your Spirit along with the agonizing pain of previous separation. Cherish that feeling. It's not about how far you can go into the pose or how long you can stay there; it's about building on the moments that you can feel connected to your Spirit while being in the pose.

ENDARKENMENT

One of the best ways to experience the physical expansion that accompanies opening to Spirit is to first experience its opposite, what I call endarkenment. This breath-squishing exercise will help you feel the consequences of how cramped, unmindful breathing starves your body and dulls your mind. It's a collapsed way of living.

To experience endarkenment, begin by sitting cross-legged on the floor and closing your eyes. Collapse your spine, curving it so your chest is closed, diaphragm squished, abdominals compressed, and back sore. Slowly raise your head so your neck kinks as if it were your seventh hour at the computer. Make your breath shallow and uneven. Think all your worst, darkest, most depressing thoughts. What's your personal fave? *I'm not good enough. I'll never have what I want. Things will never change. Life is pain and suffering.* Feel fully how this creates a smoggy, cobwebby environment inside of you. Get that these are the consequences of your collapsed thinking and collapsed body—absorb it, wallow in it; feel the straining, struggling. You can't breathe. *Life is a drag. Everything will suck forever.* Feel how this puts you into a state of hopeless despair and apathy. This is endarkenment. These are the actions that drive your Spirit out. Take a few moments to amplify the feeling.

Then sit up straight and begin to breathe, clearing out the smog and cobwebs. Offer your breath as a precious gift to nourish your Spirit. Attune to that subtle or obvious change in your energy. Don't collapse yourself back into endarkenment, but instead breathe in fresh life, fresh opportunity, the chance to live the way you really want to instead of the way you most dread.

Take a deep breath into your Spirit, feel the brightness of the life force sparkle you up inside. How many of us breathe our whole lives and never feel that? Sparkle up!

UDDIYANA IN HORSE STANCE WITH BACK TRACTION

Uddiyana, which is Sanskrit for "belly flies up," is a wonderful pose for turning on that sparkly energy. It's important to do it on an empty belly, so do it either first thing in the morning or two hours or so after eating. The benefits of Horse Stance with back traction are strength and flexibility for the legs, hips and buttocks, and healing and decompressing the low and mid spine. To begin, come into Horse Stance. Stand three feet apart, bend the knees to a right angle, align knees over heels, feet turned out slightly. Place hands on hip crease and thigh, pressing strongly to traction the back. Straighten the elbows. Inhale through your nose and exhale *forcefully* through your mouth to expel the internal smog. Stay empty of breath, pull your belly in back toward the spine and up, flaring the ribs out. Keep back straight, align shoulders over hips. Tuck your chin down toward the chest. Hold 5-10 seconds. Then relax the belly and inhale. (If you find yourself gasping, make sure to relax the belly all the way before inhaling.) Do Uddiyana three times. Deliberately inhale brightness into your core. Uddiyana stimulates and tones your abdominals and core, and gets you out of your mucky thinking.

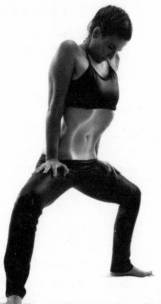

Uddiyana in Horse Stance with Back Traction

I encourage you to make your relationship with your Spirit the most passionate love affair of your life.

9

TURNING SHIT INTO FERTILIZER:
COPING WITH SETBACKS

I LAY ON MY BACK on the bed while my friend Madaline pressed her hands firmly into my torso. There was some kind of energetic clog there; I could feel it—a dark, stagnant pool deep inside me. It wouldn't move, wouldn't move, wouldn't move. Madaline was dutifully digging around my diaphragm, doing deep muscle work, trying to heal it. Then it happened:

I'm about three years old. Some guy is on top of me, squeezing me, squeezing me, squeezing me with his legs. I'm stifled, suffocating.

I sat up and pushed Madaline off me, gasping for breath, my heart beating in my throat. In that moment, I knew a truth I didn't want to know: I'd been sexually abused.

I'd long had my suspicions. Whenever I had sex, I'd often feel an intense sense of nausea, a desperate need to puke, or had to fight the urge to pass out. I'd never understood it, and it certainly never occurred to me to talk to anyone about it. Whenever clients had started telling me their own stories of sexual abuse, I'd felt a knowing beneath knowing, but it wasn't ready to come forward. Now, suddenly, it was. I also knew from my clients that people had stories behind pain. I was ready to tell my stories. "I need help," I told Madaline.

She sent me to a clinical hypnotherapist with many decades of experience named Morris Netherton, Ph.D. I remembered him from when he'd lectured at Rosalyn Bruyere's seminar. In fact, Rosalyn had suggested I see Dr. Netherton when I studied with her, but I'd blown her off. Dr. Netherton specialized in treating people with physical and emotional problems by using what he called past life regression; he'd even published a highly regarded book on the subject called *Past Lives Therapy*. I'd taken an immediate dislike to him during his lecture. I'd had enough of the airy-fairy people around me in Rosalyn's class telling me they'd been my Egyptian lover in a previous life. Puh-lease.

The next Tuesday, against my better judgment, I found myself sitting in Dr. Netherton's office on a couch amid an explosion of pillows and blankets. "What are you doing here?" Dr. Netherton asked. "I've had a few flashes," I told him, "but I don't know what they mean." I didn't understand at the time that repressed memories typically come out in exactly the kind of flashes I'd been having. He asked me fifty-four questions: What do you know about your birth? What child were you in the birth order? What drugs was your mother on when she was pregnant? How much school did you have? I'd never organized my life that way. It took me two or three intake sessions to get through them.

Dr. Netherton tried to get me to go back into my childhood, and I just flat out refused—going through it once was horrible enough, thank you. So he started explaining about past life regression. Dr. Netherton's theory was that a past life perspective was helpful to have before going into your own childhood history. I had to learn to live and die, live and die. What did the soul learn in each life? What carried forward? What are you stuck with? If you were hanged in a previous life, you might have the umbilical cord wrapped around you in your next incarnation, or you might grow a tumor in your neck. The past had lessons for the present. You didn't have to believe in this kind of spiritual evolution for it to be effective, Dr. Netherton told me. Good; I thought it was all ridiculous. But what the hell, I'd give it a try.

We started doing weekly sessions. I'd come in, sit on the couch, and Dr. Netherton would guide me. He'd first put me in a relaxed, focused state, and flashes would come.

I'm being drowned. I'm being burned to death. They're torturing me.

They're piling rocks on my chest; I'm being crushed and I can't breathe.

It always sounded ridiculous to me when I described these fragments afterward to Dr. Netherton. "I don't believe this stuff," I said. "How do I know I'm not just making it all up?" He was unfazed. "Yeah, yeah, you think you're making this up? So make up another story, right this moment." But whenever I tried doing that, it wouldn't work; something about those fragments felt true. "Don't worry about putting it all in order," Dr. Netherton told me. "It's going to come out in a messy way. It'll rearrange itself eventually. It's going to feel invalidating at first."

I didn't even have the language to describe what was happening to me. I didn't want to accept it. *Things don't happen this way,* I thought. My whole belief system was getting blown to hell, but I figured I'd just hang on and see what happened.

Extreme stubbornness seemed to follow me from one life to the next. It was embarrassing to realize that I had been an antiauthority asshole a thousand years ago, and I haven't changed. What was I not learning that I needed to come to terms with? But I was also gratified to learn that, even far back, I'd been determined to end the suffering of my people. I began to understand the difference between saving someone versus teaching that person to end his or her suffering. I began to see the beauty of my altruistic desires, even if they needed redesigning. I discovered that the definition of who I am was really vast. It stretched across millennia. It also occurred to me, *Hey, whatever I lived through as a child can't be as bad as dying four hundred times,* so that gave me the courage to crawl into my past. I told Dr. Netherton I was ready to return to my childhood.

Dr. Netherton would begin each session by finding an induction point—a bad dream, a strange phantom pain—as a way into my past. He'd have me lie down—he would never touch me—and focus on, say, a painful point in my body. "When's the first time something happened that made that pain?" he'd ask. Mostly I'd just get blanks. But gradually, I began to open up to the process. Our appointments were every Tuesday; my body started getting so used to the sessions that it would amass sensations for us to probe. "What's going on today?" Dr. Netherton would ask. "Connect to the time." I'd go numb. Then:

A blue room. A white room. A cinder block room.

I'm waking up. Where am I? Ow. Ow. Ow. Everything down there is sore and aching, everything. They've cleaned me up.

I kept hitting these blanks, blanks, blanks. I really wanted to heal, but my internal response was *No way.* I couldn't go there. I could go to any past life—the killing fields, a war zone, a cramped cockpit as a gray-suited pilot in World War II—but I wasn't ready to go to my childhood.

Dr. Netherton took it slowly. I'd tell him about some pain that kept coming up, and he'd say, "Connect with the very first time you felt this crushing sensation in your ribs." *Hmmm.*

Tree stump.

"What else do you see on the tree stump?"

Blank blank blank. *Something on my throat.* Choking.

None of it made any sense.

"We're getting information. It's okay," Dr. Netherton reassured me. "The blanks could be drugs. It could be that you were unconscious. We'll work with it until it goes." I was holding my disbelief in reserve. Memories started floating up.

I'm crawling across a mesh metal table outdoors. I'm out of my mind with hunger. I'm so desperate for food, I'll eat anything, anything. I'm reaching for the salt and pepper shakers. That's as close to food as I can get.

I'm crying, gasping hysterically.

I'm about six years old. I'm wearing a white dress with embroidered flowers. I'm so, so hungry. We're at some kind of lodge. The man is coming.

It's awful but it's finally over. The man has washed and cleaned me. I'm dressed in the white dress. He strokes me on the head. I close my eyes and relax inside. I'm telling myself, "It's over. It's over," and then the man says, "See? She enjoys it."

Piece by piece by piece, a picture was slowly emerging. Now I understood why I'd always hated white, refused to wear it. Later I learned that my abuser wouldn't let me eat unless I obeyed; no wonder I had all those flashes of gnawing, all-consuming hunger. I also learned that I'd frequently been drugged during my abuse, which is why so much of the experience was blanks, blanks, blanks.

While in therapy, I'd fallen in love with a wonderful man named John, and we were married. I would go home and tell John everything based on the pictures I got with Dr. Netherton. It was humiliating, but I wanted to break the chain of silence. John listened patiently, tears running down his face, but neither of us knew what to do with this horrifying information.

As I started to sort through more and more during my sessions with Dr. Netherton—how the numbness and drugs had been archived in my body—I began to experience even more unpleasant sensations, often a searing pain a day or two later. It was as if as soon as part of my body had learned not to be numb, it was ready to reveal another horror to me. I didn't know what to feel or believe about this, only that I understood it to be true.

Ow! Someone's cut me with some sharp object down there. It hurts so much!

At that memory, my body jumped off the couch. Later that day, I went to a salon to get waxed before a photo shoot where I'd be dressed in minimal Yoga clothing. The beautician ripped the wax off my bikini area and patted the area with a soothing cloth. She peered closely with a frown. "Where did you get this scar?" she asked. I bolted upright to look. She showed me an old hairline scar by my genitals. I had a shocking revelation: *This is true.* That realization slammed me into the next: I was still holding off the pain, betrayal, horror. *This is true. This really happened to me.*

I wasn't crazy—what was *done* to me was crazy. I had lived through that hell. Now, my fears and nightmares all made sense.

How was I supposed to live with that horrible truth? The self-loathing was a tidal wave. As a child, I'd been taught that I was despicable, that every bad thing that happened to me was my own fault. All those wrong beliefs were smacking me down over and over; I wasn't able to process them yet. The Annie who'd tried to leap to her death came back in full force. I lived in fresh, disabling terror of my abuser. It brought me back to a time when I was small, in the thrall of my crazy mother.

There were moments when that wall of loathing began to ripple. For a moment I'd be able to see a ray of sunshine without those deep layers of shame. Then the wall would slam back: strong, cold, impenetrable. I didn't know how to feel. On one level, I had a sense of great relief. On another, I felt more damaged than ever before—too damaged to live.

I talked to people who'd likewise come to terms with their sexual abuse. It helped that they didn't think I was despicable. They weren't horrified. I learned by trial and error who was good to talk to and who wasn't. People could only hear that ugly stuff for so long before they filled up. It took me a while to stop blaming them or myself for that; some had a quarter-inch capacity to listen to it, some six miles, but at a certain point, they couldn't hear any more either. That just meant I needed to be able to talk to someone else or take it into therapy. My behavior was very bulimic regarding my experience; when I got triggered and started to talk, I couldn't stop. I'd puke it out on whoever was near. John took the brunt of my terror and loathing and confusion. I pulled away from him so he couldn't pull away from me first, even though ours was a relationship I treasured.

One day Dr. Netherton and I were in a session when a particularly horrifying memory swam up out of the dark.

I'm in a cinder block cellar, a kind of holding pen, alone, cold. There's a tiny window with a glimpse of daylight. Looking out, I'm desperately wishing to be out there, but I know I'm going to be imprisoned forever. No one can help me. No one will save me.

When I left that session with all its hideous detail, I drove out into the complete filth of Pasadena. It was one of those smog alert days where the air is so disgusting it makes you want to climb into bed and pull the sheet over your head. But now I was able to celebrate being outside—the sky, the trees, the asphalt sparkling in the sunshine. I was driving home, out of that cellar. *Freedom!* I could have left completely devastated by those memories, but instead, I realized I'd survived. The little girl looking dispiritedly out that tiny window had given up that she could have a life, but my soul, my Spirit, hadn't been broken beyond repair. I was stunned by the Beauty of the world in all its stinking, smog-filled glory. *This world is amazing, and I'm in it.*

But just like the stoplights flashing red and green before me, my feelings strobed on and off. Relief/horror. *I survived/I am so tainted.* I was unfixable. How could I trust myself to live in this world and not destroy others?

Slowly, Dr. Netherton helped me come to terms with what had happened to me. Another intense memory bubbled up.

I'm maybe two or three years old. They're saying terrible things about me. Terrible things are being done to my body. Slam! My head is being smashed against something hard. The world goes black.

I'm terrified. They are filming. They're calling it a screen test. I desper-
ately want someone to rescue me, but I know that no one's coming. Shock.
Terror. Pain. I feel that woozy feeling again.

With that, Dr. Netherton had tapped what he called a keystone experience. He wondered whether those head injuries, all that physical
and mental trauma I'd been subjected to, might explain the epileptic fits,
even though I didn't even have a name for what I was experiencing until
I had that seizure on the train to Guadalajara for my Yoga training. How
many times had I woken up bleary? I was always exhausted because of
my fear of sleep, when the horrific nightmares would stalk me. When I
woke up, I'd often feel sore and achy. It wasn't unusual to find blood on
the sheets. My mouth would feel stretched and sore, my tongue sting-
ing. Had I had an epileptic fit in my sleep and bitten my tongue? Was it
oral rape? Had I been drugged while being raped? Was I bleeding from
an injury from working with the horses? All those possibilities made it
that much more difficult to discern the truth about the abuse and to get
underneath the confusion. It was frustrating—and exhausting. But that
keystone experience held out the promise that I might be able to work
through the epilepsy that still tormented me from time to time.

Back when I was living with Ganga, I'd begun to learn how to control the fits. That was hard work, but it was better than the Dilantin that
made my body clumsy and my brain smoggy. Against doctor's orders, I
went off the Dilantin and began to stalk the epilepsy. It had taken years,
but I was tired of living in victim mode. I decided that there must be
some kind of signal preceding the fits that I was missing, so I started
looking for one. I discovered that I would get particularly clumsy and
stupid right before a fit. If someone was talking to me, I'd have to focus
intently on putting the words in the sentence together, and by the time I
figured them out, the speaker would be on to the next paragraph.

When I was stupid, I was at my least resourceful. At first I panicked
at the sign of a fit—*Oh my god, it's coming*. Then I decided to reframe
things—could I win against this? At the first sign of that electrical storm
inside my head, I'd stop whatever I was doing and pull the energy out
of my head by breathing deeply, rubbing my feet, or walking. I drank
gallons of coffee, which kept me on a revved-up frequency beyond the
epilepsy's reach. The first time I succeeded at curtailing a fit, I had been

doing Yoga when I accidentally kicked the back of my head, right where my abuser had smashed it when I was a little girl. My body tried to have a fit. I could feel my essence trying to jump out of my body, but I grabbed it, like Peter Pan dragging his shadow back toward his body. It was an intense battle, back and forth, back and forth, until the electrical storm passed. I'd remained conscious, hadn't bitten myself up. I still had fits after that, but I began to get a sense that there was a part of my brain that I could keep hold of, like a tightly coiled spring that was harmless as long as I never loosened my grip.

With Dr. Netherton, I began to unwind the spring of my epilepsy. As we explored the memories of my abuse, I would have violent physical reactions as the emotions came roiling up. Dr. Netherton taught me to breathe through the anxiety. He encouraged me to track persistent tormenting thoughts so we could explore them during our sessions. If I couldn't stop thinking, *I'm just a cancerous scab on this earth,* or, *I'm 135 pounds. I deserve to die,* it was a sign that we were on the trail to something. Dr. Netherton helped me connect these traumatizing thoughts to the endless discussions I'd overheard among my abusers about my worth *and* worthlessness. I began to realize that all my beliefs that I was both too much *and* not enough came from those experiences when I was so young and helpless. Any situation that put me into that state of mind—*I'm a cancerous scab*—was a trigger. It threw my big, grown-up body into the fearful state of that young, helpless, terrified little girl. In that state of mind, I could lash out at anyone and everyone. I needed to recognize where the disabling belief came from and track it back to its source—to disarm it. Little by little, Dr. Netherton helped me work the fear out of my body.

Recognizing my triggers—and the experiences that had probably caused my epilepsy—helped me approach the disease in a new way. At a certain point, I could feel the mental hand of control on the epileptic spring in my mind; it could catch and stop the spring so that it would gently relax its loops rather than uncoiling violently like a deadly rattlesnake, triggering an epileptic fit. I began to feel a sense of ease in my brain. It was the weirdest sensation, like Pigeon pose in my head—a warm, liquid feeling as though my mind were taking a relaxing bath. Together, Dr. Netherton and I searched out the last vestiges of my epilepsy.

We worked together for years. Step by step, I became more adept at processing my own life experiences, at managing the tidal waves of self-loathing so they no longer pulled me under every time. I started to have a sex life I could relish. I began to learn to set boundaries.

After all these prolonged battles—bulimia, epilepsy, sexual abuse—I thought I'd finally cleared all the detritus from my life. At long last, my life was on an upswing. I mean, it was really good. I'd found a way to deal with every setback life could hand me and, against all odds, I was thriving.

And then—once again, damn it—I got flattened.

It was Mother's Day, in May of 1993. The day before I'd sent up one of the more unusual Mother's Day prayers: *Dear Sacred Ones: Let me please be done with my mother. Let me finish the mother cycle in my life.* The next day I was having lunch with one of my students, Trish, in a restaurant ironically called A Votre Sante (To Your Health). I shifted in my chair, and all of a sudden, I was airborne flying to the right. I had one of those magic moments in which time slowed way down, giving me a chance to think. I saw that my head was flying right toward the corner of the neighboring table. *No way,* I thought, *I am not going to deal with any more fucking brain damage.* I twisted in midair to avoid the table and miraculously landed on my feet, then turned around. "What was that?" I thought there'd been an earthquake. "I don't know," Trish said, as shocked as I was. I was totally dazed, adrenaline coursing through me. I looked down at my chair; one leg had fallen right through a rotting floorboard. The force of the chair collapsing into the floor had flung me into the air.

The next morning when I reached out to turn off my alarm clock, I discovered that my legs wouldn't work. They were paralyzed. I lay in bed completely freaked out; paralysis was one of my greatest fears. I used my arms to pull myself off the futon onto the floor, where I rubbed and beat my legs to get some feeling into them. Finally I was able to pull myself to standing and stumble downstairs, my legs giving out several times along the way and sending me crumpled to the floor.

How could I teach Yoga if I could barely move? From that moment of the chair's collapse, a whole series of bizarre circumstances began to spiral me downward. My business began falling around my head. My marriage started to collapse. I'd gone from being incredibly fit, strong, and flexible, with my business taking off, to losing almost everything I had. How could I deal with one more setback?

EAGLE LICE

A few years ago I was leading a Yoga retreat in Utah near Angels Landing. A local falconer, Martin Tyner, came to give our class a demonstration. It was thrilling. Martin unwrapped these huge cages with covers like they were presents and, one by one, extracted a falcon, a hawk, an owl. They were magnificent creatures, but I had eyes only for Bud, the gorgeous golden eagle with the fierce yellow eyes, who spent most of the lecture perched on Martin's arm.

Martin told us an amazing story about another eagle he had rehabbed. When he first found the eagle, it had a badly injured wing; without the ability to hunt, this beautiful creature would soon be dead. The eagle required very delicate, precarious surgery—so delicate, in fact, that the bird couldn't be sedated and restrained as in a normal operation. Martin would have to hold the injured bird just so for several hours while the veterinarian operated. As he was holding it, a very large eagle louse—we're talking about a half-inch long!—climbed out from the bird's feathers and began to crawl up Martin's arm, up his neck, and into his scalp right near his ear. Martin couldn't risk letting go of the bird to flick the vermin away; the eagle's life was at stake. He had no choice but to stand there, stock still, while this creepy, disgusting thing probed his scalp.

This was a huge epiphany for me: when you're going through a hard time, you've got to learn to hold on to what's precious no matter what. Hold it lightly, hold it gently—just hold it. Everything else that's going on—whether it's creepy, disgusting, annoying, or scary—is just eagle lice.

The precious eagle was what was important to Martin. For me, my connection to my Spirit, my medicine pipe, and teaching Forrest Yoga to Mend the Hoop of the People—those are my eagles. I've got to protect them no matter what crises are slapping me around. Where there are eagles, there are eagle lice. There's no way around it. Anytime I have a setback, I remind myself, *This is just eagle lice. Just hold that eagle steady so it will be able to fly again.*

SPIRITUAL FOCUS:
DISOBEY THE DICTATES OF YOUR CONDITIONING

DHARMA JOUSTS

As I explained in chapter five, a dharma joust is a way of reframing a situation to challenge yourself, asking: *What can I do differently, right now, to disobey the dictates of whatever is trying to lead my life?* It's resourceful problem solving. Making the decision to do a dharma joust doesn't mean you have all the solutions; you're just stating your intent that you're going to find them. Doing dharma jousts with the aftermath of my abuse, my bulimia, my epilepsy, and my paralysis has taught me not to give up. Whatever setbacks I face, I now know to joust with them instead of rolling over with my throat exposed and paws in the air.

There's an old joke about a boy who digs furiously in a huge pile of pony poop. The pile's taller than he is, but he just keeps shoveling away. "Why are you wasting your time digging up all that manure?" another guy asks him. "With all this shit," the boy answers, "I figure there's gotta be a pony in here somewhere." In our dream worlds—especially mine— we find the ponies in the mountains of manure. But even if we don't, the challenge becomes: *How can I take this shit and use it for fertilizer, even to find humor and beauty within despair to make beautiful things grow from it?*

What possible fertilizer could I find from having been sexually abused? My first thought was, since I've gone through this, maybe if I stand in all of this damage, I can show others that they're not alone. But I wasn't ready to go there yet. Still, there had to be something of worth I could do with my experience. I wanted to be able to cultivate desire, to say "I want ___" and feel I deserved it. I wanted to be able to stop myself from going into guilt and shame whenever I blew something. I wanted to learn how to stop making everything my problem. I wanted to stop taking myself away from help and instead ask for what I needed.

My therapy with Dr. Netherton had planted a seed of empathy and compassion for myself. I could own and respect that I had to have been pretty damn strong to have been that tiny and lived through those horrific experiences. The physical shock of being regularly drugged and raped had been a steep price tag for that knowledge, but it was proof that I was a survivor. I realized my present life problems were nowhere near that daunting—that's an amazing perspective. I still had to wrestle continually with the belief that I was too damaged to live and love. I still felt most comfortable playing the hermit at the edge of the tribe, the one who people could visit for healing and then leave in her corner. But I had found the courage to learn how to sit down and eat with people. I could walk out to the ocean in Santa Monica and see the sparkle on the waves. How could I never have seen that before? Stop. Breathe. Wait. Look. There it is. The moments of seeing something other than my damage started to lengthen; the periods of self-loathing shortened. After years of bulimia, I began to know the feeling of being able to eat something and not cramp around it or want to puke it up. How amazing to experience a meal resting in my belly. Ordinary miracles.

My dharma jousts with epilepsy have taught me not to crumple in the face of a grim prognosis. Every medical professional told me that I had this insurmountable, incurable medical condition with no hope except for surgery or drugs. Doctors warned me, "Don't tell anyone you're epileptic or you'll lose your friends." Some people even considered my epilepsy to be a sign of spiritual possession. No one told me therapy would help. My dharma joust was refusing that mind-set that nothing would change, nothing would help. I began my dance of exploration against so-called insurmountable odds, and I found openings. Working with Dr. Netherton, I had fewer and fewer fits. I haven't had one for about fifteen years, although my brain still gets reactive around flickering cameras or lights.

So this is the fertilizer: know that if you go to a doctor and he says there's no hope, you can look elsewhere. There's a great saying: "Insanity is doing the same thing over and over and expecting different results." If you want a different result, do something different! If one stream of information doesn't work for you, keep looking for what does. This is incredibly important for anyone who's ever been abused or struggled with illnesses of the immune system, such as chronic fatigue syndrome or Epstein-Barr virus syndrome. Frequently we have fought against something in our life and couldn't beat it, so we just gave up. That giving up can translate into a compromise to our immune system, to being unable to fight off viruses or illnesses. My triumph over my epilepsy has been an incredible treasure, as has been the gift of teaching others how not to give up when they receive their own difficult diagnoses.

Recovering from my paralyzing accident at the restaurant took years. The MRI showed I had a herniated disk and ripped muscles in my neck and back. John had to carry me up the stairs so I could teach at my Yoga center. He'd lay me down on a sheepskin rug because I couldn't take any hard pressure on my bones. I felt like an invalid. I hated asking for help. The stress eventually became the final blow to a marriage I treasured, which was already strained from my process of working through abuse. We ended up divorcing. My business was in tatters, and I'd lost a loving relationship.

I sent up a prayer: *No matter what, Sacred Ones, I want to finish this. Bring me what I need to do next in a gentle way, a Beauty way.* Praying for gentle was a huge leap for me! Because of my injuries, I connected with important chiropractors, and I began to receive compelling dreams on how to heal my body. Out of that, I came up with the abdominal series of Forrest Yoga, such as Abs with a Roll. I found out how to breathe into specific spots to bring life there. My healing skills grew exponentially because I had to work my way out of that injury. My Seeing skills became enhanced because I couldn't take bright light in my eyes—I would puke. The only solution was to lie down on my sheepskin with my arms over my eyes and teach. I found I could energetically see people in the back of the room and give them directions. This totally weirded my students out, of course, but it was beautiful for me: I was teaching the class by reading energy. I'd lost so much because of the chair accident, but what astonishing gifts I received in return.

Whenever you hit that place of despair, it's a red flag; you're about to step onto the battlefield for a dharma joust. Ask: *What can I do differently in this moment? How can I turn this shit into fertilizer?* You're in control here. Turning your karma to dharma means figuring out what to do with what's been done to you. Look for the gifts in your experience.

STOP PLAYING THE VICTIM

Turning your back on victimhood is an important step toward healing from setbacks. I could have decided to wallow in my abuse, epilepsy, paralysis. That might have gotten me some pity and shallow comfort, but the Brave-Hearted Path was to challenge my victimhood instead of wallowing in it.

Many of us have been victimized: we've been fired, robbed, dumped, attacked, betrayed, and more. A lot of times, it's not our bloody fault. Sometimes we blame ourselves: *If only I'd known. . . .* We're genuine victims in that moment, and it leaves a trail of trauma. Now we have a decision to make, though: turn our back on victimhood, or continue to live in a cringing way that makes us everyone's prey. The media supports victimhood; turn on the news and you're bathed in terrifying stories of unsolicited violence. Some people can get juice from being pitied or getting extra attention or help. The downside of victimhood, however, is that you live in a fearful state that keeps you from walking forward into what you want. Even more dangerous, you emit a psychic energy, a neon light that advertises, *Hey, I'm lunch—come eat me!* A predator can spot a victim faster than a social worker.

When you go into victim mode—*I'm under attack!* or *There's not enough to go around!*—your body sets chemical and hormonal cascades in motion. Cortisol, the stress hormone, floods your body. Your brain goes from rational thought to reactive red alert. The stress response wreaks havoc on your body, compromising your immune system and making you a sitting duck for chronic illness.

When I caught myself living in a fearful state, I decided to enroll in a class called Model Mugging that taught women to fight when they were attacked. We had female and male instructors. The female instructors coached us and showed us dozens of different ways to beat the crap out of the male instructors wearing heavily padded suits. When I learned to fight back, I turned my immune system back on. That's why I'm not a believer in ahimsa, the doctrine of nonviolence; we must learn how to fight for what matters to us. Our body knows how to fight and if it stops, we're dead. Before my therapy and my decision to stop being a victim, I was sick all the time. I very seldom get sick now.

Make a decision that you don't want to live as a victim. Interestingly, when you change your thinking, you short-circuit that stress response—and your body has a little temper tantrum about it. Suddenly, its old familiar coping mechanism—freaking out—isn't working. You might think that deciding not to live in victimhood will help your body calm down. And it will in the long run. Initially, however, you'll experience just the opposite!

As you begin to go through the process of working through your setback, you'll experience some (often alarming) signs that you *are* healing: rocket voyages all over the emotional spectrum, physical symptoms such as diarrhea or a runny nose—the body literally releasing useless crap. You might break out in acne or rashes—you're releasing the emotional pus balls inside of you. The symptoms may make you feel crazy, but that's just part of the process. The old balance isn't working for you anymore; the old structure has to fall apart. It's distressing unless you recognize this as a healing crisis.

Dissolution is scary! Remember the lesson from the Death Meditation: Death equals opening up space for new life. We don't equate chaos and falling apart with approaching the truth, but they are part of it! It takes a while for new patterning to form on a mental, physical, spiritual, and emotional level. Your body's chemical response to a given situation will be challenged over and over, but each time you say, "I'm going to take a stance," instead of, "I'm going to play victim," you teach your body how to heal.

Everyone's timetable for the journey from victim to victor is different. No two people will experience a healing crisis the same way. How do you know when it's over? Sometimes you just wake up and you're happy for no good reason. I recognize healing is near completion when my students start having orgasms in their sex life—or even on the mat! (They're quite happy to share this news with me.) Now that's something to look forward to!

USE TRIGGERS TO FIND YOUR TRUTH

In Forrest Yoga, we have a saying: *Never waste a good trigger.* A trigger is something that sets you off. Someone says something and you get white-hot angry or terrified out of proportion. Someone touches you lightly, and you react as though you've been attacked. Triggers are horribly uncomfortable; they put you into a state of reactivity so quickly that you're sometimes gasping for breath and wondering, *What the hell was that all about?* Yet triggers can teach you so much, even though you have to wade through the mess. They're a sure sign that something deep inside you needs healing. They're a chance to work deeply. Track the sensation. It will lead you to the emotional pus ball.

Working with Dr. Netherton taught me to connect my childhood abuse to two reactions—my quickness to anger and my tendency to plummet instantaneously into an emotional abyss. Anything I perceived as a provocation or attack would trigger me, but once I began to recognize why I reacted as I did, I could trace the hurt deep inside my body, breathe into it, and begin to heal it. Then I could return to whatever person or situation had triggered me with a fresh, clear approach. I still have moments of reactivity, but now I can do a dharma joust and spot the trigger in the moment. Then I can say, "This is my trigger; it may have been true then, but it isn't now." When I do this, sometimes my body responds instantaneously, as if my cell tissue has chemically transformed around the trigger. Triggers can be proof of your victimhood as well as an invitation to track a deeper truth.

THE LESSON OF SISIUTL

Coping with great setbacks is hard work. You often relive the horror of trauma as you revisit it in order to process it. It can be emotionally exhausting to work through triggers. The fears that can come up are formidable. I challenge my fears by calling on the power of Sisiutl, a powerful Supernatural for the Native Americans of the Pacific Northwest.

Sisiutl is terror incarnate. This hideous snake with heads at either end of its body travels on moisture—not just rivers, streams, dew, and rain, but your tears, your blood, your slick sweat. Sisiutl preys on fear. Whatever most terrorizes you, that's what calls Sisiutl to you. Wherever your terror lives, Sisiutl will tap it. In the Northwest, the trees are twisted and bent and dead because they tried in vain to run away from Sisiutl—that's what happens when you flee your fear.

When Sisiutl comes after you, the urge to flee is almost irresistible, but if you turn to run, Sisiutl will blow your soul irrevocably into the Four Directions—and that's the end of you. Your only chance of survival is to face Sisiutl. You must learn how to take a stance, get balanced, breathe deeply, keep your feet active, and do your power dance. Medicine People learn an actual dance, utter prayers of protection, and sing their Medicine Song. With every inch that Sisiutl oozes closer to you, you'll become more aware of its slimy skin, its terrifying glare, its horrible grimace with its protruding tongue, razor-sharp teeth, and fetid breath that reeks of the grave. Hold on to your faith and Spirit as Sisiutl comes closer, closer. Keep dancing and singing, stay steady, no matter how terrorized you are; Sisiutl's other head will turn toward you. Now you have two terrifying heads coming at you! In the midst of the worst of that most unimaginable terror, as Sisiutl's teeth are inches from your face, its heads will come eye to eye with each other. In that moment, it gets the gift of seeing itself, because she who sees the other side of self sees truth. Those two sets of eyes become lost in each other's stare. If you have stood bravely, Sisiutl won't bite you; instead it will slowly turn and leave, and with its departure, your terror recedes. Sisiutl leaves you with the gift of courage, heart, and faith that you can stand up against insurmountable odds. The Wisdom Keepers, called the Stlalacum, are the companions to Sisiutl; they remind us that we're irrevocably changed every time we stand up to terror.

Sisiutl is my ally. Whenever I'm completely terrorized, I know I have to do my dance and sing my song. You must learn what's necessary to do *your* dance and take *your* stance. Your dance could be simply planting your feet in the earth and refusing to be run off anymore. Get your feet active and breathe!

You'll have to dance with Sisiutl over and over again. But now you'll know how to face off against this terror. Whenever a setback threatens to crush me, I focus on Sisiutl. No matter how my knees are shaking, I sing my Medicine Song, do my dance—and I back the monster down. Until next time.

MENDING A BROKEN HEART

Whether you're a banker who wanted to be a writer, a housewife who longed for a career, or a computer programmer who wanted to act, there's heartbreak in turning away from your heart's desire. That same heartbreak finds you when you lose someone you think is irreplaceable. In an effort to protect your heart against further pain, you can close it off. I've learned that every time I risk loving, however, that act mends and strengthens my heart.

If you've been devastated by a broken heart, the healing is challenging. When that happens, you'll need to learn to love again in little increments. A man I knew was buried in grief because his wife had died. His heart was broken; he was ill and disengaged. He was filled with righteous inner dialogue for why he should stay in shutdown forever—*I was lucky enough to have the love of my life once, why ask for it again?*

I have no patience for that type of drama. Yes, you were fortunate to have your beloved. But I promise you that now you're seeing this person through rosy glasses; you're not remembering all the friction that's the normal part of a relationship, and you're being a damn fool for letting your delusions shut you off from more love. Let's say you have this exquisite gourmet meal—the best meal you've ever had, your taste buds are full and sated on every level, including a deep appreciation of the love and attention that making the meal required. Now, because you had this one great meal, which you can never have again, does that mean you shouldn't eat again? Of course not. Love is the same way. You have friends, a dog who loves you. Now warm your heart with these small hearth fires of love—the two-legged friends, four-foots, and winged friends who care about you. Cultivate these small loves.

You may want to close down your heart forever after a great hurt because you never want to experience such pain again. Your fear of heartbreak may be Sisiutl-sized. Make a Brave-Hearted choice: be touched in your heart and allow love to grow your heart braver.

PHYSICAL FOCUS

When people have been knocked flat by setbacks, I don't recommend what are called restorative Yoga classes, with their props and pillows and nice Yoga naps. Those don't change your energy. If you're shut down and your blood is pooling in your limbs, it needs to move and be cleansed with fresh oxygen. Don't wallow in victimhood—get moving on the mat!

I also like to use heat as an ally to melt the hardened places and scarred areas of your heart. When I teach classes, I make sure the room is heated to eighty or eighty-five degrees. I call this sweat lodge Yoga; it's amazing for facilitating the process of opening your heart and other shielded areas.

BLOW THE COBWEBS OUT OF YOUR HEART

Uddiyana (see page 204) tugs on your heartstrings and helps blow out the cobwebs so you can better connect with your authentic self. When you're heartbroken or scared, it's hard to feel your abdominals. With Uddiyana, you get control of your abdominals and make them work. Use your heartbreak or terror as a guide, and breathe into wherever the terror has imprisoned you. When you empty your lungs, blow out all that stuff that's keeping you stuck. When you take that inhale, it's really sweet because you've been without oxygen for a few seconds—and you'll treasure all the more the chance to breathe in fresh life, strength, and courage. Teach your abs to support your heart. I also recommend Dolphin (see page 156), Elbow to Knee (see page 58), Chest Opener on the Wall (see page 92–93), and Camel (see page 30) to open the heart.

SUN SALUTATIONS

In the old days, every time I had a setback, I'd want to "use." I'd do any kind of binge—drugs, alcohol, bulimia. As an alkie, I'd learned to punctuate everything with alcohol. Immediately afterward, I'd feel righteous vindication, but then I'd feel hideous, as if I'd been slimed.

Addiction, I now know, is really about a deep need screaming to be met. When people are in acute pain, they go to drink or drugs. We turn to addictive behaviors because they separate us from the anguished scream of that need. When we don't know how to solve something, we look to dull it. But drugs and alcohol just turn off the fire alarm, leaving the fires of destruction raging. It's much better to turn and face the pain and find out what the area needs. It needs help, a Firefighter, so help it.

Regular twelve-step programs didn't work for me. Then I found one that did: Sun Salutations. Now if I'm in pain about something and a craving to dull the pain comes up, I'll do Suns because they're so simple and if I do them out of order, it doesn't matter. I feel virtuous afterward, as if I've bathed my cells in sunlight instead of pollution. I feel lit from inside and outside, clean, open. In the grip of a devastating setback, I can do something good for myself—what a novelty!

Sun Salutations bring you skillfulness for moving your breath and energy. They'll warm up your muscles and lubricate the joints. The flow of oxygen and blood to your brain nourishes it, relaxes it, and calms down the mind's chattering. Feel the energy as Sun Salutations quicken your blood!

1 *Namaste:* Stand with your tailbone tucked down, your toes active, and your chest lifted. With hands in Namaste—palms touching in front of the chest—take a deep breath and exhale.

2 *Standing Backbend:* Inhale, reaching your arms up and back. Tucking your tailbone down, push your pubic bone forward. Telescope your ribs up while pushing your heels down.

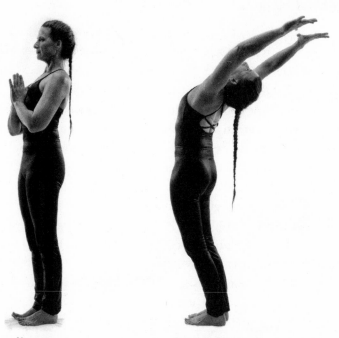

Namaste   Standing Backbend

3 *Forward Bend:* Exhale and come down into a forward bend with a straight back. Keep your neck long and feet active.

4 *Lunge:* Inhale and step your left leg back into a lunge. Sink your hips toward your front heel. Keeping your front heel flat, lift your ribs and arms. Spread your fingers and tuck your tailbone down.

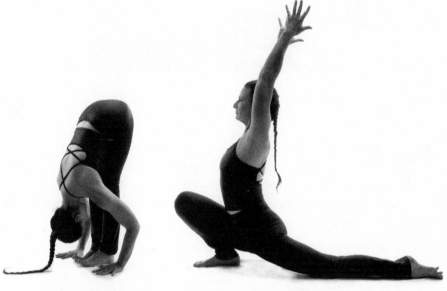

Forward Bend   Lunge

5 *Plank:* Exhale, hands down. Inhale and pull your right leg back into Plank. Squeeze your ankles together, pull your shoulders away from your ears, and tuck your tailbone down.

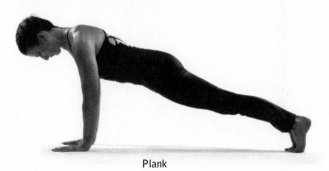

Plank

6 *Modified Chaturanga:* Exhale and place your knees down. Pull your
  shoulders away from the floor, relax your neck, and lower your torso
  to the floor.

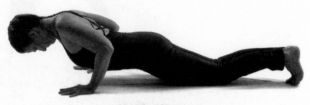

Modified Chaturanga

7 *Low Cobra:* Place your hands twelve inches in front of your shoulders. Tuck your tailbone down toward the floor. Then inhale and lift
  your torso off the floor, arching your chest forward. Telescope the
  ribs, pull your shoulder blades down, elbows bent three inches above
  the floor, and squeeze your ankles.

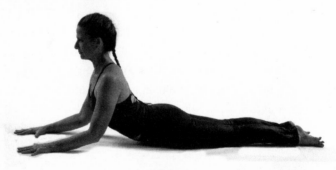

Low Cobra

8 *Down Dog:* Exhale into Down Dog, keeping your chest active. Press
  your heels down and wrap your shoulder blades toward your armpits. Press down through the web of the hand between your thumb
  and forefinger.

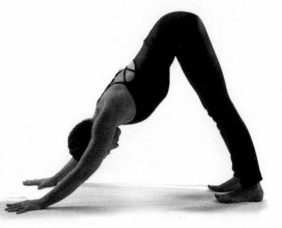

Down Dog

9 *Lunge:* Inhale and step your left foot forward into a lunge. Sink your hips toward your front heel. Keeping your front heel flat, lift your ribs and arms. Spread your fingers and tuck your tailbone down.

10 *Forward Bend:* Exhale and step into Forward Bend—legs straight, neck and torso relaxed, and feet active.

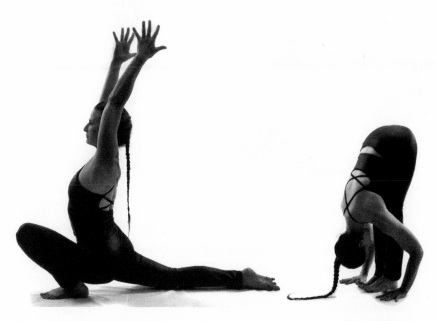

Lunge   Forward Bend

11 *Standing Backbend:* Inhale, come up with a flat back, pulling your belly in. Tuck your tailbone down and push your pubic bone forward. Telescope your ribs up and arch your back while pushing your heels down.

12 *Namaste:* Exhale with hands in Namaste. Lift your chest, keep your toes active, and tuck your tailbone down.

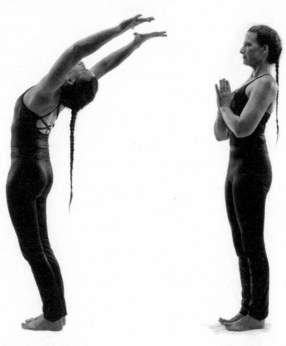

Standing Backbend   Namaste

Coping with setbacks gives us an unprecedented opportunity for evolution. Like butterflies, we can metamorphose inside the chrysalis as our lives take a new shape. We experience an incredible period of vulnerability when we emerge from the chrysalis—what I call the wet wing period—in which we face a new world where none of the old rules apply. But when we face the devastating fallout of our worst fears, and our greatest heartbreaks, we can indeed take flight. We are irrevocably transformed, freakingly beautiful.

10

THE POWER OF CEREMONY:
CREATING BALANCE AND CELEBRATING

ON MY FORTIETH birthday, my friend Madaline hosted a party for me. That was a new choice for me because I'd never celebrated that occasion before. My first forty years had been full of so much yuck and the difficult work of healing. I was glad I'd survived it, but it was nothing I wanted to commemorate. I wanted the second forty to be about celebration and thriving—years filled with respect, admiration, love.

I invited my friends and students, with one request: *Don't give me presents; give me ceremony. I want a talking circle. Tell me a story about an experience that we had together that made our connection strong.* I wanted to feed my heart.

The stories that night were amazing: tender, funny, moving. Josquin, then a fanatical vegetarian, told a hilarious story about being in my home for the first time and finding a turkey leg, stripped surgically clean, in the trash. (He didn't know I'd given it to Wicca, my parrot, a meticulous bone nibbler and polisher.) He'd shuddered; for him, it was like stumbling across a crime scene. Did he really want to keep company with such a rampant, committed carnivore? "I swallowed hard," he told all of us who'd gathered in the circle, "and decided to love Ana anyway."

Everyone in that radiant group shone a different loving light on me. It was an evening filled with roars of laughter, tears, hugs. I began rebuilding my internal foundation on a wheel of truth, love, affection, wisdom, and humor. I kept reminding myself not to shut down because there was so much sweetness, love, and affection. I felt in balance, able to design the life I'd desperately yearned for.

SITTING IN CEREMONY

Sitting in ceremony—a kind of sacred pause—helps me to take stock of where I am in life, celebrate my successes, and assess where I need to get my life in balance. Balance is still one of my biggest challenges; I balance better on my hands than I do in my life! Ceremony connects me to the Sacred Ones and to my essential self. Most typical celebrations—like the sickly sweet birthday cake with lots of presents—don't speak to me. Ceremony does.

Traditionally, Native American ceremonies weren't written down and were kept fairly secret between the Medicine Person and the participants. I believe that because we don't live in tribes with a local Medicine Person anymore, the information needs to be brought out for our people so that anyone who has a burning desire to learn can use these teachings. This is not a dishonoring of tradition. By writing my ceremonies down, it's my intent to Mend the Hoop of the People.

Most people head for ceremony when they're in trouble, just as we connect to Spirit when we're dying. Use ceremony not just to fix what's wrong, but to notice what's right and to focus on bringing more of what you want into your life. Set your intent with ceremony, and your whole life will have purpose. Paying special attention to what matters—*I want to add three things to my Beauty Report* or *I want to make my gratitude list*—brings it into being. Make ceremony a regular part of life.

Ceremony is a way to celebrate and invite Spirit in. To sit in ceremony is to make a conscious decision to step into a sacred space, to ask a specific question, and to listen for guidance from the Sacred Ones or Jesus or whomever it is you listen to. The answer we receive is usually outside of what we're expecting, so it's important to stay open so that the response can come in. It takes courage to ask for what we want because we're often taught that that's not okay.

Learning to ask the right questions, instead of waiting like a baby to be spoon-fed, is an important life skill. It's an art to ask really good, precise questions; if you ask messy questions, you get messy responses. Prayer—asking those questions—is a part of ceremony. Do you see prayer as begging or beseeching or negotiating? Who do you think you're negotiating with—the principal? Make your prayer a very clear offering. Collect your thoughts, decide what matters to you, and speak what's in your heart.

Ceremony is also a perfect time to reflect on what you have so you can be grateful for it. Focusing on gratitude changes us alchemically and moves us out of hungry-ghost mode, the state of being in which nothing is ever enough and we constantly want more. When we move into gratitude, we can acknowledge and feel the sweetness that's working in our lives.

I've created ceremonies that make sense for my life; they allow me to pause and reflect, to ask questions and receive answers. I'll share some of my ceremonies in this chapter so you can experiment with me to find out what works for you.

SPIRITUAL FOCUS:
CREATING MEANINGFUL CEREMONIES

CEREMONIES FOR EQUINOXES AND SOLSTICES

I love that everything is always changing. As the earth journeys around the sun, the days lengthen or shorten toward the solstices; in between they find moments of perfect balance, the equinoxes. As children of the earth, it's easier for us to make changes if we work consciously with the earth's changes. It's fun to look at your life through these lenses: What needs realignment? What can you put aside so you can refocus on what you want to nurture? How do you want to spend your energy? Are you moving in a good direction, or are you on auto-pilot?

Equinoxes, when day and night are equally long, are about balance. Spring Equinox is the perfect time to ask yourself: *What am I going to be planting and harvesting? What beginnings do I want to make?* Just as im-portantly—*what endings are in order; what do I not want to work with anymore? What needs balancing (work versus other aspects of life)?* Spring is a very sexy time; everything's coming up, standing up. It's a good time to start things. Six months later, during the Autumn Equinox, ask your-self: *What do I want to reap—not just eat in the moment, but harvest for my future? Am I harvesting the same old shit or something meaningful and nourishing?* Focus your intent so you'll harvest what you want.

Equinoxes are a good time to do fasts and cleanses so you can start afresh. Here I'm talking not only about cleansing yourself of poor, non-nutritious food, but also of emptying yourself of busyness, of all the nonsense that doesn't serve you. Being empty in a good way means rid-ding yourself of the toxic drains on your life force and refilling yourself with fresh energy. Then create your life with more focus and power.

The Summer Solstice is the longest day of the year. It's a playful time when you can bring more sparkle into your life. What do you need to bring into the light? I make ceremony out of the celebratory energy of the Summer Solstice. Bathe in the sun, relishing and luxuriating in the vast quantities of light that we have for that longest day.

The Winter Solstice is a time to work with the stuff of death; it's time to go willfully, deliberately, into your deepest, darkest, and most mys-terious places. What needs to be cleaned up? Where is a good restful place inside of you? The Winter Solstice is a good time to take those long sleeps, to work on your dreams and find out what they mean for your life. It's a wonderful time to ponder because there's not so much ex-ternal busyness; everything is fallow. Access, write down, and treasure the seeds of your future. Which ones do you want to nurture through the Dark Time when there's little sunlight? What will you plant for the following year? What do you want to put aside that's not worth planting again? Set your intent about where to put your life force. Do you want to pay off your mortgage? Build your Yoga practice? If you've been strug-gling with something—abuse, dishonesty, despair—do you want to con-tinue to be a victim or are you done with that? The weeds will come up as they need to, but you're no longer planting that seed. Focus on mak-ing this day the turning point in creating the life you most want to live;

write it down. On this day, it's traditional to stay up all night to pray, dance, and sing to welcome the light. After the longest night of the year, it lightens up. No matter what your night of hell or year of darkness, you can rejoice in knowing that it's going to get lighter, little by little. It doesn't matter what you believe; that is just what happens.

CEREMONY FOR DAY OF THE DEAD

I love the Latin American tradition of the Day of the Dead, November 2, when people celebrate their dead with festivities, gifts, *pan de muerto*—this gorgeous braided bread—and by cooking up all their loved ones' favorite dishes. Colorful artwork featuring skulls and skeletons is everywhere. It's a big party! People talk and laugh and reminisce. It's a time not so much for tears but for laughter, communion, and reconnection. I like to spend the Day of the Dead with my beloved dead because it helps me maintain our relationship. I don't know about you, but I never took a pact that said, "Till death do us part." I look for ways to send love and energy to my beloved dead. It's a time of renewal when I plant flowers or bushes in tribute to them. You may want to visit their grave site or a favorite place you shared with them. Tend to it—clear away weeds, plant something, or perhaps leave a cool stone or other token from someplace you both loved.

Let this be a day of treasuring. Make a simple altar. Place photos of your beloved dead on it, along with a candle. Make their favorite food and drink—to enjoy for yourself and to set on the altar too. Gather your friends or relatives and sing or tell stories—funny, sad, poignant. Share your beloved dead with your living beloveds. Do the things they would treasure. My friend Jerry and I share memories of his beloved dead wife, Doty. One time, she tied Jerry's clothes, which he'd left in disarray, into knots and tossed them onto the lawn. He'd been raised by a woman who did everything for him, and Doty wasn't into picking up after him. She made her point. He and I are still chuckling at her actions.

Even though this is meant to be a day of joy and celebration, sad, painful thoughts and tears may come. That's fine. Tears drain our wounds, which can then dry out and heal. Sit and be open to the Spirits of your beloved dead. Get quiet and open up the doors to your heart and soul and see if your beloved dead want to visit. Open up your windows so the breath of their Spirits can come in. Then wait to see what transpires.

Get your story of expectations out of the way—you don't have to experience your mother's embrace to reconnect with her Spirit. If all you get is memories or a moment of sweetness or a whiff of your mom's perfume, it's enough. The quiet contemplation of why you love this person is a beautiful honoring in and of itself. If you experience nothing else, so what? That's enough. We're so quick to judge ourselves. When we try something strange and spooky, if we don't hear or feel anything right away, we feel we've failed. If we reach out while blanketed in anguish, grief, and guilt, our beloved dead can't get through that, and neither can we. Practice setting those feelings beside you for a moment. If that's not yet possible, you may need to reach later, when the fresh rawness of your sadness has tempered. Begin with honoring your dead by feeling the love you have for each other. Relax into that.

If you don't get a heavy transmission, enjoy whatever your senses tell you. Take what happens as the truth. If nothing happens and you've had only some quiet time in repose, that's a good thing too. Just hang out with your beloved dead to the degree that you can.

SMOKING FOR BLESSING

Smoking is a basic element of most Native American ceremonies. It's the process of using smoke from smoldering sage, sweetgrass, or cedar to clean the energy of a room, object, person, or artifact, to clear out negative thoughts, bad spirits, bad feelings, or whatever else impedes clarity and healing. A lot of people use the word *smudging*, but I prefer *smoke* because I find smoke quite beautiful. When I was a smoker, I loved watching the swirling smoke float from my lips. I see clouds as smoke. Smoke is a way of tracking how the air moves—the footprints of the wind.

I like to begin my morning prayers by smoking the room. On an energetic level, smoking your environment is like taking a morning shower—it gives you a clean slate. I light a sage bundle, blow the flame out, and walk in a clockwise direction around the room to start afresh. I then call in the Four Directions, adding in a prayerful aspect and setting my intent—what an exquisite way to start the day! To learn about expanding this into a full Four Directions Ceremony, refer to www.for restyoga.com.

DREAM-TIME

I like to use ceremony to enter another sacred space where I ask for and receive information and the answer to prayers: Dream-Time. This is the Native American name for the world that opens to us while we sleep. If we prepare ourselves properly, we are more likely to receive its gifts in the form of Medicine Dreams, which are sent to help us.

Gather a notebook and pen, or audio recorder—whatever's easiest. Put a glass of water and a light beside your bed so you can see what you're writing when you wake up in the middle of the night. Before you go to sleep, drink that glass of water. The water will help fill your bladder so you'll have to wake up to pee; this makes it easier to remember your dreams and write them down in the moment. Then lie down and set your intent. You may simply want to learn from your dream, or you may want to ask for help with a specific problem through a dream that you will be able to remember. Writing down your question helps you focus on it, so feel free to do that before you fall asleep.

Whenever you wake, write down your dream *immediately,* as close as possible to when you have it—even before you get out of bed to pee. Don't worry if you can't remember your dreams at first. You'll improve with practice.

You won't necessarily recognize a Medicine Dream at first. You won't know that's what it is until you study it. Ponder your dream. What could it possibly symbolize? What does each aspect represent to you? Does this dream have any relationship to the intent that you set? *I don't know* is a perfectly good answer. You might get analytical; that's okay—it's all practice.

Start tracking your dreams. What's happening to you in Dream-Time? Is your mind digesting something that happened during the day? Go in with a curious and inquiring mind. Analyze later. Be patient and generous. Allow for learning. Navigating Dream-Time is a skill worth honing over a lifetime.

As you begin to work this, don't get too fixated on any one aspect or symbol in your dream. Everything is interconnected. Be flexible.

Let's say you've posed a very specific question for Dream-Time, e.g., *Should I leave him?* And you think you've gotten a very specific answer. Use a moon cycle—twenty-eight days—to reflect on it. Keep asking the question or any variations of it that arise. Write down whatever information you receive during Dream-Time. The question may change to *How do I get out of this relationship?* Then run it through the Chakra Process for Life Decisions Ceremony, so you're working both Dream-Time and waking time. What change will make a difference? Create a strategy, walk it, and it will flex. When you go from Dream-Time to living the dream, allow time for the full answer to form.

PHYSICAL FOCUS:
BREATHE YOUR WAY TO BETTER DECISIONS

CHAKRA PROCESS FOR LIFE DECISIONS CEREMONY

The Chakra Process for Life Decisions Ceremony is an extraordinary process to use when you want support in making a life decision, whether it is a good thing, a bad thing, or anything. If you take the time to get the information from each of your wisdom centers, you'll make a more informed decision. It is like having your own council of elders, your council of Wisdom Keepers from which to learn. It makes a huge difference if you honor the wisdom inside of you. That way you will be able to go through your decisions and changes much more gracefully and efficiently, so it doesn't have to be so damn hard all the time. The process is as follows:

1 Sit with your spine straight and breathe deeply. Settle in the core; quiet the mind.

2 Write down the issue or life decision you are focusing on today, date it.

3 Do Brahmari breathing through each chakra, as outlined on page 123.

4 Put the issue in front of you, focusing on every detail simultaneously. Get it as visceral as possible.

5 Breathe that issue into the first chakra and find out what your first

chakra feels about your issue. Write down whatever information comes up, and don't edit it.

6 Go through all seven chakras in this way. Write down each chakra's response.

7 Go back to any area that had discomfort or numbed out. Ask the area, *What do you need from me so this issue can be resolved/healed/created?*

8 Write down the action steps that you can start *today* to bring this life decision into being.

You can bring your life decision into existence with integrity and without sabotage. How great is that?

To view a more detailed description of the Chakra Process for Life Decisions and other ceremonies, refer to www.forrestyoga.com.

11

EVOLVE OR DIE:
EMBRACING CHANGE

RECENTLY I CREATED a new public Yoga demonstration. My demos are deeply meaningful to me; they're an opportunity to inspire all my students to stretch their beliefs about what's possible. This one was especially important because it was the centerpiece of a fundraiser for a cause close to my heart: yogaHOPE, which helps women who have been struggling with alcoholism, drug addiction, battery, and sexual abuse. This program teaches women how to climb out of the pit, showing them a different way of living through Yoga and sobriety.

I wanted my poses and the music that went with them to teach these women what I had learned: that if they were willing to do the work, they could build the life they wanted. They were in their twenties and thirties, yet they felt they were too old to shape their lives. Many of them were burdened with the care of too many babies, and they didn't see any open doors ahead of them. I wanted to show them: Hey, I'm in my fifties, and I can do this. In fact, the truth is I couldn't have done this demo in my thirties; I wasn't as strong, focused, or confident. I hope this demo inspires people to exceed their limitations and, when faced with a challenge, to ask the vital question, *What part of this can I do?* Build from there.

This demo was an exhilarating, challenging piece. When I first began choreographing it, I fell on my ass over and over. The moves required all the strength and balance I had, but my goal was to show them the fierce and beautiful dance of my Spirit, to inspire, to ignite hope, to dance the truth of *If I can do it, so can you.* As I fine-tuned the demo, I especially focused on honing my transitions to be as beautiful, balanced, and touching as possible. *The transitions are as important as the poses.* In fact, all of life's transitions are worth paying attention to. My goal and yours: to make them beautiful, open, and flowing, to stay centered, strong, and conscious during a transition so that whenever we arrive, we arrive with integrity. We need to reframe change, to go through it in a way we can be proud of instead of thrashing and flailing.

Evolve or die. To me, those are our choices. We either embrace change, or we die—or we might as well be dead. I trust that the changes I choose do make a difference. I'm working for my actions to spread like a cleansing wildfire over Mother Earth, fertilizing the soil and cracking open the seeds in the forest. I can Mend the Hoop of the People to the degree that I infuse the people around me with a healing that can continue to spread beyond us. To do this, I've had to embrace change. Shift happens.

CHANGE: THE ONLY CONSTANT

I'm coaching you to dance with the one constant in life: change. Do you choose stagnation or the unknown? Every choice you make can propel you toward change or keep you in the same dulling, suffocating box. Change is rebirth. When a caterpillar weaves herself into a chrysalis and undergoes metamorphosis, she emerges as a butterfly, bearing only the merest resemblance to her earlier form. Transformation can be really exciting, but we have to tolerate an incredible period of vulnerability when we emerge from the chrysalis, unfurling our very wet, very fragile wings. We discover that none of the old rules apply—not even how we nourish our new selves. Leaves don't cut it any more; only nectar will do. I've learned to recognize that with every change, I'm going to end up in new territory—whether I embrace it, shed my chrysalis, and evolve or go down kicking and screaming. I've done it both ways and the choice is clear: I like to go through my changes with some amount of elegance and balance.

Transitions don't last forever. Transition is a really special, sacred time. It's the name given to the last, most painful phase of the dilation of the cervix during childbirth. The opening to the birth canal has to widen those last two centimeters in preparation, and it's *hard work*. You can't push during this time—that's counterproductive and prolongs the labor; you just have to hang on and breathe through it. Every major life transition is like having a child—you're birthing a new piece of yourself, with its own mind and destiny. You ride that primordial wave, or you crash.

When I began writing this book, I was going through another change: divorce. I was thrashing, angry, scattered, and my actions reflected it. Then my friend, who had gone through a divorce from her husband of twenty years, gave me some really beautiful advice: "Under all the anger and all that stuff, it's important for you to reconnect to the love you had for this person that brought this marriage together in the first place as you go through the ending of it." When I embodied that, it helped my ex and me work on our dissolution so it could be finished in integrity and beauty.

In the case of divorce, it's important to grieve the death of the dream of two lives woven together. My partner and I designed and built a house together, grew certain aspects of my business together, traveled all over the world, and did really great work. I wanted to honor that. I've watched myself grieving the dream, I've felt betrayed, I've felt that my love was thrown away, and I've thought, *Okay, good, I'm done.* But just because I *declared* it done didn't mean it *was* done. I had to go through a few more spin cycles. But the more I gave myself over to each new cycle, the more quickly it went through me so I wasn't trapped in anger or sorrow or rage—it felt more like moving through wind currents. Sometimes I had to become very chameleon. One minute I was blue, then red, then yellow.

I've developed a very quirky energy around change. Once I chose to live, I had to reframe why all these weird things happen to me. I had to recognize with every change that I could either embrace it, shed my skin, and evolve—or find myself fighting stupidly to stay in the rot. I play with cultivating a sense of humor about change. I'm an emotional fan dancer right now. I do my best to keep breathing and to stay centered through it. Each time I go through what comes up, I get a little nugget of wisdom. I want to help you do the same—evolving is the best game in town!

Are you willing? If so, you'll receive wisdom from every transition. Growing older is a change that brings golden opportunities, so ponder ways to reframe growing into your wiser years. And for women, aging brings special challenges to natural cycles. The next Forrest Yoga practices help you surf change with energy and fascination.

SPIRITUAL FOCUS:
UNDERSTANDING THE CYCLE OF CHANGE

While every change is unique, its arc is predictable. The best way to embrace change is to greet it with Exercises for Evolution.

EXERCISES FOR EVOLUTION

1 *Recognize when you feel the winds of change blowing through you.* You feel something coming. Sniffing or sampling the wind, you can *smell* something coming. Instead of shutting down and going numb or getting drunk, get ready! Start your breath, get your feet active, get balanced. If you have the internal wherewithal to recognize that what you're sensing is change, ask yourself, *What else can I do right now to prepare?*

2 *Reframe change.* Stop identifying change as loss. Ask yourself, *What will I get* by changing, instead of, *What will I lose?* Then ask yourself: *How can this loss be a lightening up or an unloading?* Heartbreak, bitterness, a belief system that you're a loser—maybe you can't unload it all, but there's for sure *something* you can let go of. Search it out. What does this change call for? How can you make your transition a fun ride?

3 *Disobey the dictator.* A lot of your resistance to change is about obedience. You've grown up conditioned in myriad ways: sexuality, reli-

gion, schooling, community. It's powerfully uncomfortable to change that conditioning, but feel the effects of obeying something that is no longer worthy of your obedience. Put down those beliefs that ruin your life. Be a rebel: just disobey. Use rebellion and disobedience as catalysts for change.

I've been doing this since I was a kindergartner; I clearly remember taking a stand on my very first day of school. I'd been burning to go to what I'd fantasized as an institute of higher learning. Then, on that very first day, our teacher insisted we take naps (I wasn't tired) on our blankies (which I didn't have). I argued with the teacher: "Why should I have to sleep when I'm not tired?" "Because it's naptime." That made no sense. I disobeyed, and she sent me home labeled an unmanageable child. (No wonder waking up is such a core teaching in my work!) I just had to take radical action to challenge a belief system that creates suffering—I had to free myself.

I still free myself as often as I can. On a winter day, it was really cold in my hotel room, but a polite sign on the heating unit said, "This unit is controlled by the wall thermostat." It wasn't. Freezing, I just ripped the grid off the wall heater, discovered the real controls, and cranked that baby up.

4 *Expect the next change.* Expect the next change because it's coming. Hoops, circles, cycles. Maybe you'll have time to adjust before the next wave of change, maybe not. Embrace it—don't just brace for it. Fighting change is as stupid as fighting the seasons. You're not going to change change, but you can change how you go through it. As I came to terms with my divorce, I began to feel the tingling excitement of wondering what's next. This is how change can transform us, if we ride the currents instead of raging against them. No matter what the change, four essential elements will help you surf change instead of sink beneath it:

1 *Breath:* Use it to bring awareness to what's happening to you and to nourish yourself.

2 *Water:* Use it to nourish, cleanse, and hydrate the rivers and streams of your body.

3 *Yoga:* Use it to create the energy that will bring more strength,

flexibility, alignment, openness, and balance to your body—and to release the emotional backlog archived in your body. I call this being a "life athlete."

4 *Meditation:* Use the quality of your attention and silence to look and listen within. This is an opportunity to wake up and listen to the desires of your Spirit. Start with that!

Implementing these four basic elements on a regular basis can help you elevate and sustain your mental, spiritual, emotional, and physical health. When you begin to reframe the opportunities within change, you give yourself another perspective and a broader understanding of the choices available to you. Are you doing what's most beneficial in terms of honoring yourself and your truth? If you don't like your choices, break out and go after what you most deeply desire. When confronted with a difficult choice, ask yourself, *Does this brighten or dim my Spirit?* Make a Warrior's Choice. Get brilliant.

CEREMONY OF RELEASE AND LETTING GO

Change is often difficult because we have trouble letting go of the past. I use a special ceremony when I go through the process of change: the Ceremony of Release and Letting Go. It has two parts: recapitulation, the process of digesting the experience; then a physical action and pranayama to help cleanse the experience.

Divorce. Moving. Leaving a job. Ending a friendship. Closing a business. A beloved's death. Getting married. Becoming a parent. These changes can be cataclysms in our lives, even when they're positive events. They can bring up a lot of baggage, and if we don't take the opportunity to sort through it, we'll just drag it right into the next phase of our lives. Recapitulation isn't only about release; it's also about reevaluating and digesting an experience, pulling the wisdom out of it. Sometimes you don't know what you've gotten out of an experience until you've moved the crap out of the way to take a closer look.

Not every change requires you to work through the process of recapitulation. If a change in your life doesn't call up a lot of issues, then you don't need to go through this exercise. But if you feel yourself thrashing around because you're fighting a change, unable to move forward cleanly and clearly because all your old stuff is holding you back, it's worth doing this ceremony.

Doing the recapitulation process can take fifteen minutes to several hours—it's up to you and how quickly you can release the wasted hours or months of following an obsession. Recapitulation leaves you feeling clean and clear because you're taking physical actions as well as emotional actions. Pranayama will always reset you in a clearer, more powerful place. Examining your beliefs is like taking sharp pieces of shrapnel out of your soul and heart, and there's healing from that if you give it adequate time and conscious action. These sensitive areas need careful tending to prevent more scar tissue.

At first, when I thought about losing my marriage and my partner, I fell into a black pit of terror. I used the Ceremony of Release and Letting Go to sort it all out. Was I terrified that I couldn't feed myself? Nope, not a problem. Was I terrified that I couldn't pay the bills? Nope, not a problem. Was I terrified that I wouldn't be able to work? Nope, I had all that in place. As I walked my way through it, I realized that this terror I was experiencing didn't really track; it wasn't my authentic experience. I felt sorrow and rage, yes; terror, no. So whose terror was this?

I had to walk down a long, black tunnel until I found myself back in my mother's uterus. When my mom had been pregnant with me, she was on her own at the time and she didn't have a way to feed herself or pay the bills. The terror I was feeling was really hers. Here was my mother, a woman with two other small children, pregnant with a third, alone (my father was out of the picture then) with few saleable skills, and no means of support—is that not every woman's nightmare? Well, almost; it certainly was hers, but it wasn't mine. With that insight, my terror went away. I also found myself clinging, holding, clinging, holding. That led to another false belief I needed to excavate—that the only way I could exist was if I was married to my man. The more I poked at that, the clearer it became that holding on to some fantasy or socialized belief that wasn't happening was a kind of death. As I peeled back all these emotions, resolved them, and came to terms with my divorce, I began to feel a bright new energy.

To begin the process of recapitulation, identify whatever issues are coming up because of a change you're going through—divorce, job loss, etc. Imagine each issue—e.g., trust, abandonment, self-worth, and the like—as a separate web. Each web contains all the feelings, thoughts, and beliefs you have about that issue—all the what-ifs. If you're going through a divorce, for example, some of your individual webs might be: *What if I grow old alone? What if no one thinks I'm desirable ever again? What if I open my heart again and someone stomps on it?* Remember, even joyful prospects, like marriages, can have sticky strands: *What if I'm not good enough? What if I hate his family or they hate me? What if our religions clash?* Picture these what-ifs as individual strands of the web; any one can send tremors through the whole structure.

The next step is to choose a single strand of the web and investigate whether that belief is really true for you. If not, can you release it so you can move forward? For example, suppose you're going through a hor-rific breakup with your beloved because he cheated on you. You might have webs for each issue such as trust, fear of betrayal, blame, and the like. Now it's time to go through each strand of each web one at a time and test how true each of those beliefs is for you. What are your core beliefs about each strand, where did you learn them, and are they still true for you today?

For example, if your beloved cheated on you and you now have trou-ble with trust, your what-ifs might be: *What if I can't trust myself to make new connections? What if I can no longer put my faith in other re-lationships because I can't trust those people anymore either?* Where did you learn your first lessons about betrayal? Who taught them to you—parents, friends, lovers? Did your dog die when you were little and your parents didn't tell you? Did your parents' divorce break your trust? Did a friend lie to you? Follow the strands to the origin of the belief. Feel how far back your current trigger resonates within your strand of belief. Your concerns about trust may be legitimate, or they may be based on decades-old beliefs that were specific to circumstances that are no lon-ger relevant.

Examining the web of your beliefs can be time-consuming because we often have very complicated feelings around change. For example, when I had to close down Forrest Yoga Circle, my Yoga studio, I wres-tled with sadness, loss, anger, betrayal, and fears of losing my practice, my community, my sanctuary. My feelings of betrayal led to trust issues, so I had to carefully comb through my past and review what my parents had taught me about trust, what I'd learned about it from lovers and peers. Only after I thoroughly investigated that strand could I move on to the others. The recapitulation ceremony was so valuable to me that I did it as my final gift to my Forrest Yoga Circle community. It was the closing and final ceremony of Forrest Yoga Circle.

As you examine the origins of each feeling in each strand of the web, ask yourself: *Is this fear real? Am I holding on to a belief I created when I was younger that no longer serves me? Is this really true for me now? If not, am I ready to let go of this belief so I can live more authentically?*

When you've determined that you're ready to let go of a belief that no longer serves you, follow this thought work with physical action and pranayama to cleanse the web.

Begin this part of the ceremony by lighting a candle; bringing in the fire element helps.

1 Sit in front of the flame and close your eyes. Get centered. (You'll keep your eyes closed throughout this ceremony so you won't get dizzy.)

2 Focus on the web of the issue you want to work with.

3 Picture placing *one* aspect of the issue/strand of the web at a time on your left, beside you. Don't try to do more than one at a time or it won't work.

4 Turn your head to the left and inhale the one strand that you placed there.

5 Hold your breath.

6 Turn your head from left to right, back and forth, back and forth, until you feel the need to exhale. (Turning your head—which of course turns your eyes—helps uproot the issue and scramble the old programming.)

7 Bring your head back to center. Exhale and *release* your false beliefs about that issue into the candle flame. Use the fire to burn what you want to cleanse from your life. Set the intent that the belief will no longer have a hold on you. Pledge to not give in to it.

8 Now pick the next strand and place it to the left.

9 Inhale and repeat the process until nothing else comes up or until it's time to move to the next topic.

Go through one whole web this way. As you're working each strand, other details or sub-strands may come up. Work those too, all under the main aspect. Let the ceremony take you wherever it needs to go, and re-capitulate whatever needs to be released. Sometimes it takes more than one session to finish a web.

DINOSAUR BONES

Sometimes you can put heart and soul into recapitulating something and yet it won't release its hold on you. I did everything I could to clear up everything around my poisonous mother. I finally got to a dead end; I just couldn't get rid of the remaining murderous hatred. So I did what I call an Einstein. Einstein took a huge problem—why is the speed of light constant?—and instead of trying to solve it, simply declared that he'd just take it as a given, and he came up with $E = mc^2$, making something beautiful and useful out of an insoluble puzzle.

So I did an Einstein on my hatred for my mother. I decided, well, I can't get rid of this petrified poison, so I'm going to use it to build something awesome. I felt these crystallized mounds of crap radiating toxicity inside me. I decided they were like ribs, the big bones of a dinosaur. I used them in an internal way to build the roof and walls of a beautiful cathedral that houses something deeply meaningful to me: my ethics. My ethics govern how I am in the world, how I move with integrity, honesty, love, compassion. If you can't get rid of something, recycle it. I've built my ethics to be the opposite of what my mother represents to me.

What I didn't know was that those great arching ribs of my internal cathedral weren't sealed; the toxic sludge was leaking. This petrified hatred had leached into the rest of my life, giving me an unconscious hatred of women—including myself because I am a woman. Then something completely surprising happened that stripped away that invisible curtain. I began a romantic relationship with a woman, one that required me to face all my issues and ethics. Where did this person, this relationship—all of it so foreign to me—belong in my life? In order to love this person authentically, I had to blow up my internal cathedral, the entire paradigm of beliefs and ethics about what's appropriate, my capacity to love, and more. That action deeply pulverized those dinosaur bones of crystallized toxicity and hatred.

That relationship broke my heart. After I ended it, I received an invitation from an amazing musician and medicine singer, Susan Osborn. "Come sing with me," she said.

"I'm not a singer," I told her. But she insisted that I was. So I went. And while I was singing for her, singing purely from my heart, I had the most intense vision. I could see my own broken heart, cracked and crazed, with an intensely brilliant starlight radiating from its jagged seams. The light was like a star nova. Internally, I began to push the broken shards away; beneath them was another heart, emanating this glorious bright silver-white light.

What a gift for me to find that brilliance underneath the cracks of my heartbreak. Suddenly the vision shifted, and I saw myself standing in a burnt-out forest of ash. As I watched, the ash was absorbed into the ground and fresh green growing things were slowly starting to pop up. Above me, vultures—the peace eagles—were circling. I was flooded with a sense of peace and completion.

My burnt-out relationship and my broken heart left me with a true treasure amid a maelstrom of change. My hatred of myself as a woman had collapsed, dissolving the meanness and self-mutilation. Now I have an internal openness and space I've never had.

GROWING INTO OUR WISDOM

When I look in the mirror these days, I can see my skin doing its aging thing, and I think, *I've lived a very intense life, and my face reflects it.* But I don't look at getting older as a bad thing. I look forward to the next achievement. I get a really big kick out of creating and practicing these intensely difficult demos. It's taken me a lifetime to develop the strength, conditioning, and concentration, and to open the lines of energy going through me. I want to make the most of these!

I'm wiser these days. Traditional Native Americans believe that at a certain age, around fifty-five to sixty, you have an opportunity to become the Wisdom Keeper of the tribe—a holder of the history, stories, and survival skills of a full life; that's a rich resource for the people of the tribe. As we age, we have another Warrior's Choice, either to purify and become a Wisdom Keeper or to continue to hold on to a lifetime of poison and become a toxic old hag.

Our culture fixates on the young; we undervalue the precious, hard-earned gems of a full life. It's up to us, the Crone Collective, to change this by living differently from what is expected of us. How fun is that? We can inspire each other, our young people, and ourselves by being a living example of potential actualized. Imagine being a passionate, vital person, knowing you have something of value to contribute. Make the choice to model a different, much more enticing future for our young people rather than allowing yourself to be ignored and devalued because you're over a certain age. We can embody and model the beauty of a rich spirit versus just a wrinkle-free face. Challenge yourself to learn something at least once a week. What new interest sounds delicious to explore? Perhaps a new concept or insight into yourself, or a new Yoga pose? As you get more adept, reach for learning something daily.

The older we get, the less room we have for indulgence in bad habits. The consequences of our actions become readily apparent. If we eat poorly, act poorly, think poorly, it's easier for us to discern—and therefore easier for us to make the decision to change. The aging process has much to do with the cells slowly dying from oxygen deprivation and toxicity from dehydration. Breathe more! Drink more water! Active Yoga, deep breathing, and sweating all help to cleanse the cells and revitalize them. The quality of your life will profoundly change. Do this for yourself; you're worth it!

SURFING THE CHANGE OF WOMEN'S NATURAL CYCLES

Lots of women come to me because of difficulty with menopause: hot flashes, erratic moods, brain blanking. If this is your situation, I want to help you reframe it: what old garbage can you allow to be swept into that cyclone so that when you emerge, you can synthesize all your life experiences and begin to glean the wisdom from them? You've lived this long; you've learned *something*. Moon pause—as my Native American teachers call menopause—is a really wonderful time because it's the physiological induction point for ceremony—when you come out, will you be a candidate for Wisdom Keeper or just a burden to your people? What can you do during this time to be a gift to your people?

There's a profoundly negative, degrading attitude in our culture regarding physical, mental, and emotional issues. Our society takes perfectly natural events and casts them as sicknesses we need to overcome. This attitude is particularly true when it comes to our natural female cycles: moon time (menstruation), pregnancy, perimenopause, and moon pause. These negative attitudes definitely don't promote healing, and you don't have to buy into them.

I cherished the ceremonies I learned on the rez. Native Americans long ago developed ceremonies as a way of honoring women and encouraging them to embrace each new stage of life as a celebration and an opportunity for growth. In traditional Native American societies, women would move to the women's lodge for the full time of their moon cycles (five to seven days)—thirteen times a year—where they'd learn from the more experienced women of the tribe, including the Wisdom Keepers. It was an opportunity to look within, a time to learn about themselves and the mysteries of being a woman, a quiet time to honor, a time for earthy sex education (the women talked!) while being freed from their daily responsibilities.

Today's woman hasn't yet learned to honor her cycles and mysteries with a women's lodge. Our culture treats women's natural cycles as though they are a disorder or disease. Let's reframe the way we think about our cycles, which contain the elements of our own unique magic. Let's embrace them as treasures of discovery. Initiation into the women's lodge is a time to recognize and hone our intuition, to familiarize ourselves with our natural cycles. We learn to use these cycles to transform our experiences into healing medicine instead of viewing them as inconvenient annoyances.

During our moon time, our hormones can cause us so much physical and emotional discomfort. We can swing from one emotional or physical extreme to another while feeling betrayed and completely out of control. We either overqualify these emotions with righteous indignation and anger, or we completely disqualify them with remorse and grief, thinking we're ridiculous. Either way, we can easily get snagged in self-mutilating thoughts—*I feel fat. I'm all bloated. Everything's pissing me off.* What else throws you into these patterns: not enough sleep, lousy sex, sugar, too much coffee? Our behaviors have roots. Stay alert to spot what actions create what consequences.

During the time of our moon, we can begin to observe the ways we might regard ourselves, our condition, and others in contemptible terms through our speech, actions, and thoughts. We can make the choice to stop this form of self-mutilation. Rather than fighting your bitchiness, can you reframe this as a time when the gauzy veils between you and the truth are very thin? Honor that your truth and bullshit detectors are more highly sensitive. Instead of trying to be nice through gritted teeth, clamping down internally, and eventually exploding, can you use this time of heightened perception to begin to Speak Truth with grace? (I suggest doing some Lunges with Lion's Breath first—see page 91).

At this time of thin veils, one way of working with the feelings of frustration, irritation, and lack of tolerance is to understand that your usual layered and shielded self is almost naked. Also, you're in the fullness of the gathering time—the waters are backed up against the dam. Of course you feel full. This is natural and not worth fighting against. Don't allow your frustration with your body to grow. Do some Yoga, especially Elbow to Knee (see page 58). As you bleed, you release.

It's also very helpful to carve a small niche of quiet alone time. Create a simple ceremony to honor your time in woman's mysteries instead of cursing about being on the rag. Turn off the phones and television for the night, light a candle, and massage your belly with some oil in a circular motion (going down the left side, moving up on the right side). Then move on to your breasts and armpits to help the circulation in the mammary and lymph glands. If it feels good, massage your hands and feet. Now sit quietly, breathing into your womb, listening, feeling, and observing what appears. Journaling can be helpful and insightful too, especially after some silent time. It is your sacred time. Experiment. You may discover that there is power or gentleness, grace, deep inside. Is it possible to respond honestly yet gracefully to the world instead of viciously or from a shut-down place? As you get more skillful at this, you won't need to nuke the people around you. In moments of emotional difficulty, ask yourself, *What is the most honoring, truthful, and kindest action I can do for myself right now?*

We particularly need to reframe how we think about menopause, a stage of life fraught with fear, ignorance, suspicion, and degradation. We can suffer and blunder our way through, drugging ourselves senseless and adding to the archaic beliefs that women are ornamental, irritable, our worth shallowly measured by our ability to satisfy men's needs or to birth and raise children. Or we can step through the gates, explore our mysteries, burst through the chrysalis, and unfold our wings. This can be an exciting time of cultivating and growing our wisdom. Do you choose fear and diminishment of yourself, or do you choose to explore the mystery and unknown aspects of yourself? Do you choose to grow or to rot?

Once I identified my perimenopausal symptoms, I chose to move through my panic and fear about losing my mind and to reframe my relationship to my symptoms. I asked myself, *How can I use this life change? What do I need to get rid of in my life?* What a rich question! *What memory programming do I need to let go of? Who and what do I need to clear out of my life?* With the help of my acupuncturist, using wild yam cream, eating healthy, drinking more water, doing lots of Yoga, staying grounded, keeping my feet active, and making an extra effort to feel the earth with my feet, I made good use of this time. As I continued to move the things out of my life that were throwing me into a fog, the fog cleared. This is a great opportunity for you to move some fog makers out of your life. Look at the usual suspects—sugar, tobacco, alcohol, overeating, drugs, parasitic people. Is it time to say goodbye to them?

PHYSICAL FOCUS:
SURFING CHANGE

MOVE IT!

It's tempting to curl into a fetal ball when a change knocks us down. But in fact, this is the time of life when we most need to get our blood moving. When you're stuck—physically, emotionally, spiritually, there's nothing like Sun Salutations (see page 223) to shake out the cobwebs. Connecting each pose and transition by breath is a great physical metaphor for connecting your life experiences. Whatever comes, know that you can just keep breathing through it.

As I said before, emotions have to be in motion to be healthy. (Notice the word *motion* in *emotion*.) If they sit and get stashed in the cell tissue, that's when they morph into emotional pus balls. When you're processing a difficult emotional situation, Yoga can be powerful medicine. When I was divorcing, I tried to focus on the loving feelings that had once joined me to my husband so we could dissolve our marriage in the same harmony with which we'd entered into it. Of course, I didn't always succeed. Honestly, from time to time, I had those feelings of wanting to disembowel him. When that happened, I had to do something physical—get on my mat and do Lunges with Lion's Breath or Handstand, or put on some really rowdy music and stomp around and dance. If I didn't give those negative feelings an outlet, they'd turn to poison. If you want to release those archived emotions, move!

Forget Yoga naps; you need to sweat, get your bones strong, move that body around! Hot flashes are a cleansing thing—*use* the power surges. Work out and sweat at least once a day—you need the cellular cleansing. What's the big deal if you have to change your shirt a few times?

While we're at it, let's *celebrate* those hot flashes! You can go into distress and shame, or you can ride that wave of energy! You can reframe this experience by using it as a call to step into sacred mindfulness and ceremony—your own personal sweat lodge! You can use these moments as a personal wake-up call. *Wake up!* Something *powerful* is happening!

Hot flashes are a great time to burn karma. I heat my Yoga rooms so that my students can discover exciting new depths in their practice. You can produce that powerful heat yourself! Use this changing time (before it passes) to access and study your old behaviors, to sweat out what no longer works and what isn't authentically you, to sweat out the poisons and toxins you have accumulated in your lifetime, and to let go of old hatreds and resentments. Breathe out the old energies that don't serve you; inhale deeply to draw in the energy you want to live in your cells: brightness, courage, passion, aliveness, love, compassion, creativity, peace. The more you use your hot flashes, the more skillful you'll become in transforming energy, thus your life. This can be a breakthrough time. Learn to work authentically, more honestly. Tune in to your energy flows and blocks, feel how they pattern your neuromusculature, and then apply breath and your poses to the areas that need help. Work smarter with daily consistency, not necessarily less, as some doctors recommend.

SINGING, DRUMMING, AND CHANTING

We need to make noise when we make change; it moves our energy and lifts our Spirits. Doing your dance and singing your song are attributes of the Southwest on the medicine wheel; they are an integral part of who we are. In olden times, everybody sang and danced, no matter how old or cracked they were. We have lost that. We leave the dancing, drumming, and singing to the dancers, drummers, and singers when in fact we all benefit by doing these. It's about expression of self—and that's always worth doing. When you have all that guilt and grief and crap clogging you up and you attempt to resonate your voice from your heart, it moves stuff around and opens you up, and that can feel amazing.

So sing! If your critical inner voice starts its rap—*You sound like a sick dog*—keep singing anyway. I almost quit Medicine training—something so dear to my Spirit—because one of the requirements was that I had to find a Medicine Song and sing it in front of people. I hit the I-can't wall with a splat. But when I turned to run away, it ripped my heart because I didn't want to leave Medicine or my Spirit. I recognized that it would be wrong action. I had to circle back around and school myself in how to sing and chant. Now it's an ecstatic, powerful way for me to communicate.

Sing until you feel full or empty or changed. Move those stuck emotions. Give voice to your heart, Spirit, longing, grief. Even if your voice is scratched or broken, singing gives that part of you a voice, and that is healing and empowering. It can also be wicked fun.

Chanting is another powerful way to give voice to your heart. Some of my favorites are "May All People Walk in Beauty" by Chenoa Egawa and Alex Turtle, the eagle chant, "Cherokee Morning Song" by Walela, "Cree Morning Song" and "Wishi Ta: The River Song" by Sean Porter. You can download some of these songs from www.forrestyoga.com so you can sing along or chant the words out loud. You can also make a chant up; try simply saying the word *free* over and over, either as a spoken word or to a simple melody of your own devising. Feel the power of these words as they flow through your body.

I'm self-taught on the frame drum. For years I've drummed for my students in ceremony and while chanting. I recently began taking drumming lessons. I was lucky enough to fall in with Michael Metzler, a fourth-generation bell maker and one of Europe's great master percussionists. I've been studying in earnest now. Sometimes that sad old song will start up in my head—*I have no rhythm and yet I'm sitting with one of the great drummers of Europe*—and I will have to gently tell it to get the hell out of my life. My drumming isn't about mastery; it's about making a joyful noise, finding a way to express myself. Judgment has no place here. Give expressing yourself a shot. Grab an overturned pot and a wooden spoon and have at it! Drumming is yet another way to celebrate change and express the heartbeat of your life. Collect and treasure all the ways you can do this!

Learning how to play with change in a way that delights you makes life way more compelling and fun. Become a life athlete instead of looking simply toward building a career. We crave adventure. We crave fun. We crave trials that take us to our deepest depths. Surfing change is how we get those treasures.

Surfing the change wave has brought me to a wonderful new place. I have a thriving business with Forrest Yoga teachers all over the world. I'm publishing this book. I have students I adore, and I get to travel to new countries every year. And I have a really surprising and exciting new love at age fifty-four.

Get out of your dungeon and ride those dragons!

AFTERWORD:
THE BRAID OF THREE TRUTHS

THE MISSION of Forrest Yoga is to create in each of us a sense of free-dom, a connection to our Spirit, and the courage to walk as our Spirit dictates, thus doing our part in Mending the Hoop of the People. In keeping with my personal vision of Mending the Hoop of the People, this book has been around the world twice while I've been writing it. It's been to Europe, Hong Kong, and all over the United States. How fitting that it's done all that traveling with me. Eventually, it will travel without me doing the work of Mending the Hoop of the People.

Allow me to leave you with a Daily Diet for the Evolving Soul, a list of Sadhanas—spiritual guidelines—to follow each day.

- Allow time for silence, time to digest. Also make time to do your own version of your Medicine Song and Dance to quicken your blood.

- Do frequent dharma jousts by doing something previously impossi-ble to you.

- Speak the truth from a place of honesty and integrity. When you hit the shy wall, don't give up; speak your truth and open another doorway.

- Learn to work honestly at your edges. This helps you develop effective tools to deal with fear, struggle, and breakthroughs. This allows integrity, self-awareness, and playful curiosity to become part of your daily life.

- Avoid self-mutilating thoughts. Practice treating yourself with loving-kindness for an entire twenty-four-hour day, *no matter what comes up*. Extend this practice for two days, then three days, and so on.

- Practice being your wiser self in all things: when you're with your family, eating a meal, interacting with a friend, spending time with your lover, making love. Allow your wiser self to guide you in doing all these things.

- Play on the ecstatic spectrum; do things that give you contentment, joy, pleasure, ecstasy.

- Practice using sound to express your emotion, heart, and Spirit, and dance it out for the sheer pleasure of it. How? By moving in any which way.

- Practice being struggle-free. Can you find a struggle-free Yoga pose, a struggle-free class, a struggle-free morning? Explore how else you can function day-to-day besides struggling. I have learned so much about struggle in writing this book. Because of my own prejudices against the computer and other electronic devices, I've struggled. In the process, I've made the lives of everyone helping me much more difficult. Now I'm attempting to give up the struggle and instead build a friendly relationship with my computer. I'm finding that there are ways to use this little smart-stupid box to answer the ten million questions about the cosmos that I have on a daily basis. I'm not there yet, but the possibilities are so compelling that they're pulling me forward.

- Build up your strength. Doing Forrest Yoga builds flexibility, intelligence, and strength while helping you deepen the relationship with your authentic self. Accessing your intuition—the voice of your Spirit—builds personal strength and ushers integrity into your daily interactions with all beings. Have a blast with this!

A final gift to yourself: using three treasured truths of your life, build a three-corded braid through your core. The first cord is feeling the truth that you are loved. The second is feeling that you have the capacity to create love for another. The third is feeling gratitude for whatever you have in your life.

Do this now. Breathe deeply and steadily. Relax fully, feeling the support of the earth beneath you. Now connect to a time in your life when you felt without a doubt that you were loved. Breathe that in and feed it to your core. Breathe in the truth that you're loved and feed it to your cell tissue. Now, forming a shining cord of energy built on this truth that you are loved, attach it to the top of the inside of your skull and run it all the way through your core and down to the bottom of your pelvis, right where your genitals are. Brighten it up with your breath. Take a few more deep breaths.

Now connect to a time when you felt love for another, when you felt that exquisite energy of love and affection and care welling up inside of you and pouring out into another person or pet or perhaps your deep love and affection for the land. Connect to that feeling right now. Breathe deeply, amp up your breath, and pour the truth that you can love through all your cell tissue. Taking another very deep breath, form that energy that you just made into a second shining cord and attach it to the top of the inside of your skull all the way through your core down to the first chakra. Breathe on it and brighten it up.

Deepen your breath. Now focus on the last time you felt gratitude. It could be gratitude for something you have learned from this book, for example, the new and fun tools that you've learned. It could be gratitude for deep breaths, for the ones you love and who love you, or for discovering your truths and giving them room to grow into bigger truths. It could be gratitude for connecting to your heart and Spirit, or beginning the journey to do that. Or gratitude for learning how to do a Beauty Report, or drinking in the beauty of a rainbow with all your senses. Perhaps by now you're even generous of heart enough to have gratitude for the really difficult lessons in your life that have forced you to discover other parts of you. Whatever you have gratitude for, generate that energy right now. Breathe that in and wash it through your core. Offer that gratitude, like a precious gift, to feed your cell tissue. Create a third shining cord and attach it to the top of the inside of your skull alongside the other two cords, all the way through your core down to the first chakra.

Use your breath to make these three cords brilliant. Picture using your hands to braid them together: the truth that you are loved, the truth that you can generate the exquisite energy of love, and the truth that you have much to be grateful for. Breathe, and sparkle up your braid.

When you feel the winds of change blowing through you, reconnect to this braid, re-creating it as necessary. You are loved. You can love. Your gratitudes. Stay centered on feeling the truths of your shining braid. *It's yours. No one can take the truth of this from you.* Find out what nourishes your Spirit. Find out what delights your Spirit. Do something to nourish and delight your Spirit every day, even if it's for just a few moments. Consume only that which nourishes your body and soul. Give your Spirit the space it needs to grow. If you don't have contact with your Spirit yet, breathe in a way that welcomes your Spirit home. This way you can go through changes with a new balance and integrity, in a way that you're proud of.

May you grow the strength, wisdom, and courage to go deeper, find your truth, and take these gifts you have earned beyond the mat into the rest of your life. I offer you congratulations and encouragement. I am grateful to *you* for the honor of allowing me to guide you on this path. Aho. May we all walk in Beauty.

Ana Tiger Forrest

For more information on Ana's teachings and the Forrest Education Library, please visit www.forrestyoga.com.

ACKNOWLEDGMENTS

I HAVE A Spirit that is willing to break into freedom out of tradition and does so with the intent of Mending the Hoop of the People.

I am incredibly grateful to Chenoa Egawa and Alex Turtle. I had been praying for a Medicine teacher, and I got two: Alex and Chenoa came in strongly and adopted me as their sister. I am so grateful for that. Now they are teaching the Forrest Yoga Mentor Teachers, which means that they will help me to continue to weave more of the Medicine component into the Hoop. Chenoa embodies how to sing from heart and Spirit.

Chenoa, Alex, and Kelley Rush (friend, Forrest Yoga teacher, co-mentor liaison, codirector of the Assistant Program, ceremony sister, and she who kicks the door), and Madaline Blau especially have been teaching me a whole new meaning of family.

Special thanks to Panther Cat (Catherine) Allen for tracking changes through cyberspace.

A special acknowledgment to Betsy (Elizabeth) Rapoport, who helped me find my way onto the page in the same honest and fierce way I live my life. She made all the difference in the world. While we had many a hilarious argument over my profanities, Betsy spotted me and midwifed this book with love, attention, and her own brand of mama bear fierceness.

A special thank you and namaste to Linda Loewenthal; literary agent extraordinaire. She has seen the magic of my book, and felt it's purpose even before it was born. Linda has guided me like a doula thru the publishing process with skill, love and sardonic wisdom. Her unflagging stance thru the long nights of creation and edits brought me and my book through into daylight and new maturity.

To the elements—wind, fire, water, earth, storms, thunder, lightning, and rainbows—and to the Wild Ones and Supernaturals, who dance with me by invitation and whenever they please.

Aho!

Shyayla has spoken.

INDEX OF POSES